African
Woman's Guide to
a Healthy Heart

The

African-American Woman's Guide to a Healthy Heart

Editor	Anne L. Taylor, M.D.
Co-editor	Toni Branford, M.D.
Contributors	Jennifer Campbell, DrPH, MHSA, CHES
	Monica Colvin-Adams, M.D.
	LaShonda Jackson, B.S.
	Kweli Rashied-Walker, M.P.H.
	Hollis Underwood, M.D.

Association of Black Cardiologists
Center for Women's Health

Hilton Publishing Company   Roscoe, IL

Published by Hilton Publishing Company, Inc.
PO Box 737
Roscoe, IL 61073
815-885-1070
www.hiltonpub.com

Contact the center for women's health of the Association of Black Cardiologists at
abcardio.org, 678–302–4246

Notice: The information in this book is true and complete to the best of the
authors' and publisher's knowledge. This book is intended only as an information reference and should not replace, countermand, or conflict with the advice
given to readers by their physicians. The authors and publisher disclaim all lia-
bility in connection with the specific personal use of any and all information
provided in this book.

Publisher's Cataloging-in-Publication
(Provided by Quality Books, Inc.)

The African American woman's guide to a healthy heart / editor, Anne L. Taylor ;
   co-editor, Toni Branford ; contributors, Jennifer Campbell . . . [et al.].
     p. cm.
     Includes index.
     ISBN 0-9716067-6-5

     1. Heart—Diseases—Prevention—Popular works. 2. Cardiovascular system—
Diseases—Prevention—Popular works. 3. Heart diseases in women—Popular
works. 4. African American women—Diseases. I. Taylor, Anne L. II. Branford,
Toni. III. Campbell, Jennifer (Jennifer B.)

RC682.A39 2004   616.1'2'0082
                                               QBI04-200155

Printed and bound in the United States of America

"Study after study has shown that there is no effective development strategy in which women do not play a central role. When women are fully involved, families are healthier. They are better fed. Income, savings, and reinvestment go up. And what is true of families is true of communities and eventually of whole countries."

—Kofi Annan, United Nations Secretary General,
N.Y. Times, December 29, 2002

"Next to God, we are indebted to women, first for life itself, and then for making it worth living."

—Mary McLeod Bethune

"Children deserve to know their grandparents so they will become GREAT grandparents."

—Association of Black Cardiologists

Contents

PART II

Negotiating the Health Care System

APPENDICES

PART I

General Concepts

HEART DISEASE AND STROKE IN AFRICAN AMERICAN WOMEN

A t forty-nine years of age, Valerie S. lives a hectic but happy life. Valerie is a talented and creative grade school teacher in a large inner-city school. She's had the satisfaction of positively influencing the lives of many children, some of whom are terribly needy. Although she loves her work, her classes have become large, she can't always get the resources she needs to do the best for her students, and she finds that she doesn't have as much time for individual students as she used to have.

Still, her life is good. Besides having a job she knows is right for her, Valerie is happily married, with three children—two difficult teenagers and a very sweet ten year-old. Valerie's husband, George, owns a growing small business that requires long hours of work. He and Valerie don't always see as much of each other as they'd like.

The first sign of trouble for Valerie appeared when she saw her internist about a bad case of bronchitis. The doctor noticed that her blood pressure was a little high and that she had gained twenty-seven pounds since her last visit. Her lab work showed a "touch of sugar."

Valerie promised the doctor and herself that she would work at losing weight, and follow-up on her blood pressure and blood sugar.

With the best of intentions, Valerie joined a local Y. But after three or four trips to the gym, the responsibilities of her job and her family made her forget that her own health was key to everything she wanted for her loved ones. Time moved so swiftly that two years passed past without Valerie returning to the gym. And then, one day, time almost stopped.

At four A.M., one early winter morning, Valerie woke up feeling very ill. She had trouble breathing and her chest hurt terribly. She thought it was just a bit of indigestion, so she got up to get a drink of water. She remembers the glass of water, but nothing after that—that is, not until she woke up in an intensive care unit with her family gathered anxiously around her.

Valerie had had a heart attack. Fortunately, her husband's quick call to 911 and her son's CPR training, which he'd learned as a lifeguard, saved her life.

Now it was the doctors' job to get Valerie past the crisis and on to recovery. At the hospital, Valerie had a procedure (called angioplasty) done to open the closed blood vessel in her heart that had caused her heart attack. Because of the doctor's quick intervention, very little permanent damage was done to her heart.

While Valerie recovered, she felt glad to be alive. Four weeks after the procedure, on a fine, spring Sunday morning, Valerie was having her coffee on the front porch. That moment was perfect for reflection, and that led her to a question: "Why should a young, active woman like me have a heart attack?"

Valerie's story ended happily—she recovered and, most importantly, learned why she, like many other African American women, was at high risk for heart attack and stroke, and what she needed to do to maintain her good health now that it had returned. Valerie learned what she needed to do in order to lessen the risk of another cardiovascular event and to stay on the path that leads to a longer, healthier life.

Valerie's story also illustrates a terribly important point: not enough women, and certainly not enough African American women, understand their risk for heart disease and stroke, how their heart and blood vessels work or what makes them work well or badly.

Not enough women, and certainly not enough African American women, understand their risk for heart disease and stroke, how their heart and blood vessels work or what makes them work well or badly

This book gives you the information you need to decrease your risk, and your family's risk, of heart disease and stroke.

You will learn:

- How your heart and blood vessels work
- How to stay healthy if you don't have cardiovascular disease
- How to recover and to improve your health if you already have had heart disease or stroke
- How to prevent subsequent heart disease or strokes.
- How to help your family live a heart-healthy life.

The book is divided into three sections. Part I will tell you how your heart and blood vessels work. It will also teach you what happens when a heart attack, stroke or heart failure occurs.

Part II tells you what things increase your risk of heart attack, stroke or heart failure and how you can decrease your risk. The second section also teaches you why our children are at risk and what we can do about it.

Part III of *The African-American Woman's Guide to a Healthy Heart* shows you how to work more comfortably and efficiently with health care providers and with the health system itself. It will also teach you how to enter into a health partnership with your doctor or primary care provider. In other words, how to take your health in your own hands.

Dealing with the health care system also means understanding how your insurance plan works and knowing what to do if it *isn't* working. Part III guides you through that sometimes complicated path.

In the back of the book, the appendices give you:

- A yearly heart health checklist for you and your family. The list will guide you and your family through a heart health maintenance schedule. It tells you how to stay healthy day by day and how often to get the most important heart disease screening tests.
- A list of questions to ask your doctor to help you understand your heart disease and stroke risk.
- A list of resources that will guide you to further knowledge on specific heart health topics.

Maybe all this sounds like a tall order. Well, let's look at the alternative. African American women have a life expectancy six years shorter than majority women. The main reason for those too early deaths is cardiovascular disease, meaning disease of the heart and stroke. Heart disease is the number-one cause of death and disability for women, and for African American women, the risk of death from heart disease is nearly two-thirds greater than for women of other ethnicities!

Unfortunately, most African American women don't know this. A recent American Heart Association poll asked women what they considered to be their major health threat. Sixty-one percent identified cancer as their major health concern, while only seven percent identified heart disease. These women were guided by health perceptions, not health facts. The facts are that nearly one in two women die from heart disease, and that twice as many women die from heart disease and stroke than die of all the cancers combined.

Twice as many women die from heart disease and stroke than die of all cancers combined.

African American women are at higher risk for death and disability from heart disease and stroke than any other ethnic group. They also get these diseases at younger ages, and are 69% more likely to die from them, thus robbing families of mothers, grandmothers, daughters, and sisters.

Wanting to live the long healthy life every woman deserves, and wanting to protect the health of families are the best reasons I know for reading this book. So let's begin—the lessons aren't too hard and the rewards are great.

CHAPTER 1

HEART, BRAIN AND BLOOD VESSELS
What's Normal, What Can Go Wrong

Your heart is a muscle, an *amazing* muscle, that works continuously from a few months before you're born until the end of your life. The heart works by rhythmically squeezing and relaxing. In that way, it continuously pumps blood to every part of your body.

In order to do its work, the heart contains several specialized parts: valves, blood vessels and pacemaker cells. *Valves* open and close in a well timed, synchronized fashion to keep blood flowing in the right direction. The heart's own blood vessels (*arteries and veins*) supply the heart with oxygen and nutrients (food) and remove toxins (poisons) that accumulate as the heart works. *Pacemaker* cells are special parts of the heart that provide rhythmic electrical impulses that stimulate the muscular pumping contraction of the heart.

There are four chambers in the heart—two *atria* at the top and two *ventricles* at the bottom. The atria function as receiving chambers for blood, while the ventricles are the chambers that pump blood. Because the ventricles do the hardest work, the muscle in the ventricles is thicker and stronger than the muscle in the atria.

The heart is also divided into right and left sides, with one atrium and one ventricle on each side. The job of the right side of the heart is to get blood to the lungs, where it picks up oxygen; while the job of the left side of the heart is to pump that oxygenated blood out to the rest of the organs of the body. Along the way, blood picks up nutrients from the intestines, where food has been broken down into nutritional elements, and delivers both oxygen and nutrients to all the body's organs.

Let's follow the circulation of the blood from the moment when blood in the lungs picks up oxygen. This newly oxygenated blood drains into the left atrium, where it passes through a valve (the *mitral valve*) into the left ventricle (the pumping chamber on the left side of the heart).

The left ventricle pumps oxygenated blood out across another valve (the *aortic valve*) to the body through blood vessels called *arteries*.

When the oxygen and nutrients have been extracted by the organs, which use them as energy, blood is drained from the organs by another kind of blood vessel (*veins*), and travels back to the right side of the heart, where the blood is received by the right atrium. The blood then passes through a valve (the *tricuspid valve*) into the right ventricle. This un-oxygenated blood is then pumped through the *pulmonary* valve into the lungs, where the cycle begins again.

In this way, blood circulates continuously in a one-way path through the lungs and body, constantly supplying oxygen and nutrients, constantly removing toxins. The ventricles supply the

Heart, Brain and Blood Vessels

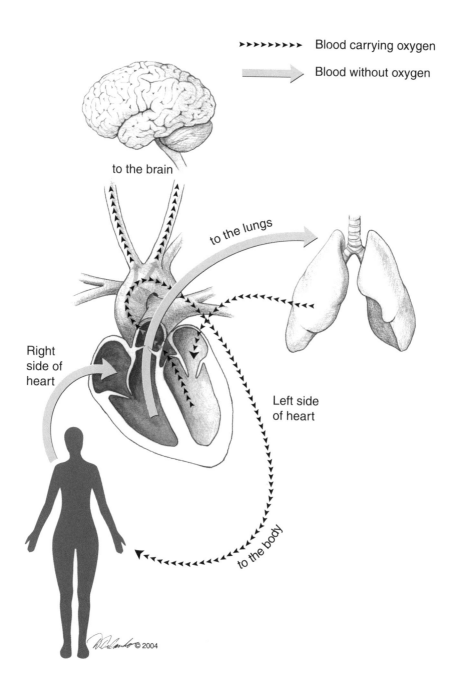

Blood carrying oxygen

Blood without oxygen

to the brain

to the lungs

Right side of heart

Left side of heart

to the body

© 2004

force (contraction) to keep blood moving; this force is felt as a heart beat, or pulse. The valves open and close with such perfect timing that blood always travels in the correct direction.

This wonderfully organized system, circulating blood to provide oxygen and nutrients and then removing toxins, sustains us through every second of our lives.

Your heart can rapidly increase or decrease the amount of blood it sends out, to meet the body's needs when you're active or when you're inactive. For example, if you quickly dash across a room to catch up with a runaway toddler, your heart rate and blood flow increase instantly to meet this need. When you snuggle into a chair for a lazy afternoon with a good book, your heart rate and blood flow decrease appropriately.

One of the most important organs the blood serves is the brain. Like the heart, the brain works continuously whether you are awake or asleep. The brain requires a constant supply of blood and nutrients as well as removal of toxins. A large, well-organized network of blood vessels ensures the brain's needs are met.

Although the heart, blood vessels, and brain are robust organs that normally work without interruption throughout our lives, they can be permanently damaged in several ways:

- Cholesterol and other cells and materials can build up in the wall of the arteries and can completely block those arteries. When this happens there is a loss of blood supply to the heart and brain, which results in heart attacks and strokes.
- High blood pressure can cause the heart to work too hard, then dangerously enlarge, and, finally, fail.

- High blood pressure, diabetes, high cholesterol, smoking, physical inactivity, can all contribute to the development of cholesterol blockages in the blood vessels of the heart and brain by damaging the lining of the blood vessels.
- Certain substances—alcohol, for example—are poisonous to the heart and can damage the heart muscle, causing heart failure.
- Viruses can attack the heart muscle, resulting in heart failure.

It's your job, working with your health care provider, to do as much as you can to prevent these things from happening to you and anyone in your family. To put into practice good heart disease and stroke prevention, knowledge is key. In the next chapter you'll learn what happens if you do have a heart attack or stroke.

CHAPTER 2

How Heart Attacks
and Strokes Happen

H eart attacks and strokes happen when blood flow to the heart and brain is cut off. This occurs most commonly when cholesterol, a yellow fatty substance, builds up in the blood vessels that supply the heart and brain with blood. Where cholesterol builds up, other elements accumulate, such as excess cells usually found within the blood vessel wall, cells that cause inflammation and finally cells that cause blood clots to form. This combination of elements that interferes with the blood flow is called a *plaque*, and it

> *Heart attacks and strokes happen when blood flow to the heart and brain is cut off.*

will eventually block the artery so completely that there is no blood flow to an area of the heart or brain that normally is nourished by the blocked artery.

Heart muscle deprived of blood flow begins to die within 10–15 minutes. Brain cells begin to die in even less time (6–10 minutes). If blood flow to a particular area of the heart isn't quickly restored, that area dies and is replaced by scar tissue. The scarred areas of the heart can no longer pump. That's why the pumping efficiency of the heart is decreased after a heart attack.

The risk of death in the early stages of a heart attack is quite high. Usually, the cause of death is a heart rhythm abnormality, which occurs when heart cells are starved for oxygen and nutrients. In this situation the regular, rhythmic contractions of the heart are replaced by very rapid, chaotic contractions. Because these rapid contractions do not circulate blood efficiently, death can result if the problem is not quickly corrected.

After a heart attack, a woman may be unable to care for her family, to dance, work, or shop. The family may suffer unwelcome lifestyle changes because of lost income. Astonishingly, that is what happens to far too many. Of the nearly 500,000 heart attacks that occur each year, about half occur in women and more than 9000 heart attacks occur in women less than forty-five years old.

STROKE

Serious trouble can also come when blood flow to the brain is blocked by plaque. When this happens, brain cells die and a stroke occurs. Strokes can also happen in two other ways:

1. Small blood clots that have formed in the heart break off, travel to the brain, and suddenly block the blood vessels that nourish the brain
2. Blood vessels in the brain, which have been damaged by high blood pressure or cholesterol plaque can burst

suddenly, depriving brain matter of the blood and nutrients it constantly needs

At the same time, healthy brain cells are killed by the pressure that builds up when bleeding occurs in a space contained by the hard, bony skull. These brain cells die very quickly and can never be replaced.

Stroke is a particular risk for women with high blood pressure and diabetes.

Stroke is a particular risk for women with high blood pressure and diabetes. You've seen the tragic results of stroke. Women who have had strokes may lose the ability to use one side of their body, lose speech or vision. Stroke is the second leading cause of disability in women and more women than men die from stroke overall. Strokes are particularly tragic because patients who have had a stroke can have memory loss, personality changes, depression, and be unable to communicate. Strokes can take away the "personhood" of those we love.

Yes, these descriptions are grim, but they show why it's so urgent that you and women in general learn how to decrease the risk of heart attacks and strokes. Heart attacks and strokes *are* preventable. All that's required is knowledge, commitment, and action on your part. The reward will be longer and better lives for you and for those you love.

CHAPTER 3

HEART FAILURE
What It Is and How It's Managed

Heart failure occurs when extensive damage to the heart muscle has taken place so that the heart can no longer pump blood efficiently enough to meet the body's needs. Damage can be caused by:

- Heart attack, which results in scar tissue replacing heart muscle
- Uncontrolled high blood pressure, which causes the heart to work harder, enlarge and then fail.
- Leaky or too tight heart valves, which cause the heart to work harder, enlarge and then fail.
- Diabetes mellitus
- Excessive alcohol consumption
- Viruses, which damage the heart muscle
- Inherited heart muscle diseases
- Vitamin and nutritional deficiencies
- Pregnancy

Heart failure affects 5,000,000 Americans each year. It is the leading cause of admission to the hospital and the second leading cause of visits to medical clinics. A common form of heart failure is "congestive heart failure," which happens when the heart becomes enlarged and weak because of damage to heart tissue. When this occurs, the heart can no longer efficiently work as a pump. As a result, patients with heart failure experience:

- Fatigue
- Shortness of breath
- Fluid accumulation in the lungs
- Fluid accumulation in the ankles, legs and abdomen.
- Heart rhythm abnormalities

The most common causes of heart failure are heart attacks and high blood pressure. Valvular disease, viral illnesses, diabetes, alcohol and drug abuse can also cause heart failure. Sometime, though rarely, damage to the heart muscle can be inherited. In women, heart failure may occur with pregnancy.

SIGNS AND SYMPTOMS

People with heart failure usually feel tired or short-winded while doing activities they easily performed in the past. They may also develop swelling in the ankles or legs. As heart failure progresses, a person may develop nausea, lack of appetite, abdominal discomfort, or a feeling of fullness soon after eating a meal.

Diagnosis

If your doctor suspects that you have heart failure, he or she will order an *echocardiogram*. An echocardiogram is a test of the heart that allows doctors to visualize, or "see", the various structures of the heart as they work. This test determines how well the heart and heart valves are functioning, whether the heart is enlarged or has areas of scarring from previous heart attacks. In addition to the echocardiogram, doctors and technicians will do other tests to find out if you have heart failure. A chest X-ray lets the medical team see if the heart is enlarged and if there's a fluid build-up in the lungs. Blood tests will be performed to look at important components of the blood, such as potassium and sodium, and to get information about kidney function. A new blood test, called BNP, aids in the diagnosis of heart failure since this substance is found in high levels in the blood when the heart is failing.

Electrocardiograms (EKG) remain the most common test to evaluate the heart's electrical system for abnormal heart rhythms. The EKG may also provide clues about the cause of heart failure.

Finding the Cause

Once a diagnosis of heart failure has been made, the physician needs to figure out what caused the failure. The two most common causes are uncontrolled high blood pressure and previous heart attacks. The usual tests needed to determine if you have blocked arteries (coronary artery disease) are the *stress test* and the *angiogram*.

A stress test is a screening test. You will be asked to either exercise on a treadmill or bicycle, or you will be given medication to increase your heart rate. Once a certain heart rate is achieved, the heart is imaged either with an echocardiogram or a nuclear scan to assess the heart's response to exercise.

An angiogram is a more invasive test in which the physician, in order to visualize blockages, injects dye into the heart's blood vessels through a small tube placed in the heart.

Managing heart failure requires a team approach with a lot of patient education and participation. The heart failure management team usually consists of the patient, nurse, educators and managers (to help the patient understand symptoms and medications), dieticians (to help patients learn how to prepare and eat appropriate foods), and finally, the physician, who oversees all of these management strategies and prescribes the appropriate medications.

While there is no medical cure for heart failure, through a combination of lifestyle changes *and* medicine, heart failure can be managed. Occasionally, surgery is also needed if the cause of heart failure is leakage of the heart valves or blockage of the arteries that nourish the heart. For patients with very severe heart failure, the only solutions may be a mechanical assist device, which helps support the heart's pumping action, or a heart transplant.

CHAPTER 4

WARNING SYMPTOMS OF HEART DISEASE AND TESTS YOUR DOCTOR MAY DO

Women need to understand the symptoms of heart disease and stroke because recognizing these symptoms can save your life, or the life of a loved one, by ensuring that you, or they, get the prompt medical attention needed. The symptoms of heart disease and stroke are shown in the tables below.

The most common heart complaint is pain or discomfort in the chest. This discomfort can range from mild, such as an ache or "nagging sensation," to severe, such as, "heavy weight," "an elephant sitting on my chest," or "a hot poker in the chest."

The chest pain of heart disease usually occurs in the center of the chest, under the breastbone. It can be severe or it may feel like nothing worse than a squeezing or pressure sensation. It may move to the shoulders, arms or jaw, or it may occur just beneath the breast bone and feel like burning or severe indigestion.

Indigestion-like symptoms caused by heart disease may occur with exertion and get better with rest. They may also be accom-

Symptoms of Heart Disease

- Chest pain alone or associated with pain in the arm, neck or jaw.
- Nausea
- Shortness of breath on exertion or when lying down
- Fatigue on exertion or unusual fatigue
- Dizziness or fainting
- Ankle swelling
- Sensation of missed heart beats or rapid heart beats (palpitations)
- Sleep disturbances

Symptoms of Stroke

- Weakness on one side of the body or one limb, or one side of the face
- Changes in vision in one or both eyes
- Difficulty either finding words or speaking clearly
- Difficulty with balance
- Sudden severe headache
- Fainting

panied by shortness of breath, sweating, nausea, or a sense of impending doom.

Heart pain may also be experienced as jaw pain, or a toothache or as a weakness or ache in the left arm, or as nausea, heavy sweating, or shortness of the breath, unusual fatigue or episodic sleep disturbances.

Chest pain from heart disease is also called *"angina pectoris,"* which means chest pain in Latin. Angina (and all of the other symptoms above) occurs when the heart muscle doesn't get its needed blood supply. If blood vessels to your heart become narrowed because of partial blockage by cholesterol buildup, your heart may not get all the oxygen needed during stressful times or times of physical exertion, thus causing symptoms with emotional stress or exertion.

The symptoms a person experiences are the heart's response to lack of oxygen. Symptoms that occur while you're exerting yourself or feeling stress, and that go away when you rest, need to be looked at promptly and carefully by your doctor. It may be a sign of heart disease.

At later stages of the disease, the arteries of the heart narrow severely, and delivery of oxygen is extremely reduced even at rest. Pain or other symptoms that occur at rest are very serious and require urgent medical attention.

Typical heart symptoms for a man may not be typical for a woman.

Typical heart symptoms for a man may not be typical for a woman. Not only can symptoms of coronary heart disease occur at a later age in women, but women may experience a wide range of more subtle symptoms including severe fatigue, sleep disturbances and shortness of breath. While some women experience the "typical" symptom of chest pain radiating down the left arm, other women have "atypical" symptoms , which may be misdiagnosed as panic attack, indigestion or flu.

Shortness of breath is an important symptom of heart disease. Often, shortness of breath occurs when you are exerting yourself and then gets better with rest. Shortness of breath occurs because the heart is unable to efficiently work if its arteries are blocked and its muscle is starved for oxygen and nutrients.

If a person is experiencing actual heart failure, shortness of breath may be constant, even when the person is at rest. Because short-windedness may also be due to lung disease or other illnesses, a physician's evaluation is needed to determine its cause and best treatment.

Fainting or lightheadedness can also be a sign of heart disease. The condition is caused by heart rhythm disturbances that occur when the heart is deprived of blood and nutrients.

All the symptoms of stroke result from loss of blood supply to the brain in areas controlling certain functions of the body. Thus, a stroke victim may feel:

- Weakness on one side of the body or in a limb or on one side of the face
- Difficulty speaking or difficulty understanding words
- Sudden blindness in one or both eyes
- Difficulty with balance
- Sudden, severe headache
- Fainting

These symptoms indicate loss of blood to the portion of the brain controlling the particular function. When the symptoms are temporary, they are called *transient ischemic attacks*, or stroke warnings. This simply means blood flow to the brain was temporarily impaired but returned before permanent damage was done.

These transient ischemic attacks or "warning strokes" are very serious symptoms. If left untreated, they may progress to permanent damage. If you experience any of these symptoms, go to the nearest emergency room to get urgent evaluation and treatment.

A special kind of stroke occurs when a blood vessel in the brain ruptures. (This is called a "hemorrhagic stroke" or "intracerebral hemorrhage," both of which mean bleeding into the brain tissue). Because the brain is encased in the skull, when bleeding occurs, there is swelling of the brain and pressure build-up occurs. This pressure build-up destroys brain tissue and may kill rapidly. Even with emergency medical attention, the death rate from hemmorhagic stroke is high because brain tissue is delicate and easily destroyed by such pressure.

A person experiencing a hemorrhage in the brain will feel a sudden, severe headache, often accompanied by loss of consciousness. This is a medical emergency and the time it takes to get treatment often determines whether the individual lives or dies.

In summary, women need to understand the main symptoms of heart disease and stroke and to seek urgent medical attention should they experience any of these symptoms. Such symptoms may, in fact, be the result of less serious illness, but it is better to be evaluated by a professional than to try to second-guess and hope for the best.

Tests Your Doctor May Do

When a woman has any of the symptoms of heart disease, her doctor will want to do certain tests to determine whether or not the symptoms are really the warning signs of serious heart problems.

Initial diagnosis begins with a thorough history and physical examination. Then your doctor may order one or more of the tests listed in Table 1.

Table 1. **Heart Disease Tests**

1. Electrocardiogram
2. Exercise stress testing
3. Echocardiogram
4. Exercise echocardiogram
5. Exercise Nuclear Scan (thallium or sestamibi)
6. Holter monitoring
7. Cardiac catheterization or angiogram
8. Electrophysiology testing

Each of these tests has a specific purpose, and evaluates a specific heart function. The *electrocardiogram* gives the doctor a snapshot of the cardiac rhythm and may also show areas of previous heart attacks or heart enlargement from high blood pressure. If the electrocardiogram is done when you are having chest pain, it may show whether you are having heart pain. The EKG may be normal even in the presence of significant blockages of the arteries, so if the doctor is still suspicious that heart disease is causing symptoms, the doctor may order a *stress test*. During a stress test, the patient is asked exercise on a treadmill or bicycle. The exercise gets progressively harder as the test goes on. The electrocardiogram is monitored continuously and abnormalities are looked for as the heart is made to work harder (stressed!) by exercise. More information is provided if some form of heart imaging is done during exercise. The two most common forms of imaging are the *echocardiogram* and the *nuclear scan*.

An *echocardiogram* is an ultrasound picture of the heart. It uses the same technology (very high frequency sound waves) to make a picture of the heart as an obstetrician uses to make a picture of an unborn baby. Echocardiograms done when the patient is at rest show the structure of the heart, how well it pumps and whether blood flow is going in the normal directions in the heart. When an echocardiogram is done along with a stress test, the doctor can see whether the heart function gets worse with exercise. If it does get worse, it is an indication that the patient has heart disease.

Another way of taking pictures of the heart is to inject a small amount of a harmless radioactive substance (thallium or sestamibi nuclear scan) into the vein, and then track with a special camera where the substance goes in the heart. A *nuclear cardiac scan* test maps blood flow in the heart and will tell the doctor if some areas of the heart are not well supplied by blood. This test is also combined with exercise testing in order to understand whether or not the heart gets adequate blood flow during times of greater activity.

Frequently, a woman may be unable to exercise due to bone and joint problems, age, obesity or simply being out of shape from lack of exercise. In these instances, a drug (dobutamine or adenosine) that simulates the effect of exercise on the heart by increasing heart rate and work or tracking blood distribution in the heart (thallium and sestamibi), may be given and the EKG and an echocardiogram or nuclear scan may be done to evaluate the heart's response to stress. These tests are called *dobutamine stress echo* or *adenosine nuclear scan*.

If these tests are abnormal, or your doctor is still not sure whether heart disease is present, she may order a *heart catheterization* or *angiogram*. In this test, the doctor places a thin tube into the blood vessels of the leg, threads the tube through the blood vessels, up to the heart. The doctor can then measure the pressures in the heart or inject a dye, which shows up on X-rays, into the blood vessels supplying the heart with blood and nutrients. This method allows the doctor to see if there are narrowings in the arteries, how tight the narrowings might be and determine which arteries are affected. If the narrow spots are positioned in a certain way, an *angioplasty* may be done to open the narrowing or a *stent* (a metal cage) may be placed in the artery to keep it open. Thus the angiogram is a test to closely and directly look at the blood vessels in the heart and potentially open up narrowings in those vessels.

If the doctor thinks that abnormalities in heart rhythm are the problem, she may start testing with an ECG, and then order a *Holter monitor*, a device that continually records the heart rhythm for 24 to 48 hours. If this test doesn't answer the question, an event monitor is given to the patient for one month. An event monitor is a wristwatch-type device activated by the patient when she has symptoms of heart disease. The device then records the heart rhythm during the time those symptoms occur. In this way, the doctor can determine the exact nature of the rhythm (that is, whether the heart is beating too slow, too fast or irregularly) as well as if heart rhythm abnormalities are causing the patient's symptoms.

Finally, if there is still suspicion that a serious heart rhythm abnormality is present, or if the patient has had very serious symptoms, such as sudden collapse, requiring resuscitation or shocks to the heart to get back a normal rhythm an *electrophysiology* test may be ordered.

During an electrophysiology test, the patient has special wires placed in the heart that can stimulate abnormal electrical activity in the heart and identify the part of the heart causing the rhythm abnormality. While this sounds dangerous, it is done in a very controlled environment with personnel and equipment present to instantly treat any abnormal rhythms which might occur.

This chapter gives you a quick summary to help you understand some of the common tests used when symptoms of heart disease are present. Remember though: ask your doctor to explain, in language you understand, any tests she recommends as well as the risks and benefits of the tests. Your doctor should provide patient education materials in your primary language, if English is not your first language. Even though some tests may seem a bit scary, they provide essential information to help you receive the best possible treatment.

CHAPTER 5

AN OVERVIEW OF
HEART DISEASE AND
STROKE RISK FACTORS

T he conditions that put African American women at risk
for heart disease are:

- high blood pressure
- diabetes
- high cholesterol
- overweight or obesity
- tobacco use
- menopause
- age
- physical inactivity

If you have any of these, *you* are at risk for heart disease or
stroke. The good news is that many of these risk factors can be
changed, so risk is decreased. Other risk factors such as age
(forty-five for men, fifty-five for women), being African-
American, family history, and for women having completed

Changeable Risk Factors	Unchangeable Risk Factors
High blood pressure	Age
High cholesterol	Family history
Diabetes	Menopause
Tobacco use	African American ethnicity
Obesity	
Physical Inactivity	

menopause cannot be changed. What's important is that there are more *changeable* risk factors than unchangeable risk factors. (Table 1)

So age, ethnicity, and family history aren't destiny. There *are* changes you can make in your own life that will make it far less likely that you will develop heart disease, or that will help you recover if you do have it. Those changes are:

- Quit smoking and avoid environmental smoke
- Exercising regularly
- Lose weight if you are overweight according to the table on p. 79
- Eating a heart-healthy, low-fat diet.
- Getting regular checks of blood sugar and treatment if diabetes is present
- Making sure blood pressure is checked regularly and controlled if high
- Making sure cholesterol is checked and controlled if high

Of the changes you can and should make to protect your health, quitting smoking is essential. Smoking speeds up the development of cholesterol plaque in the arteries of the heart, brain, kidneys and limbs by damaging the lining of blood vessels. This means that smoking encourages the thickening and hardening of the arteries. Smoking also increases blood pressure and restricts the amount of oxygen the blood supplies to the body. High blood pressure increases the heart's workload, causing the heart to enlarge and weaken over time.

> *Of the changes you can and should make to protect your health, quitting smoking is essential.*

Not only does smoking help cause heart disease, heart attacks, and stroke, but smokers who have had a heart attack are more likely to die and to die suddenly (within an hour) than nonsmokers. Smoking also increases the risk of other serious diseases, such as cancer and osteoporosis (brittle bones in women). Women who smoke have premature aging of the skin. Asthma and ear infections are frequent in children exposed to smoke in the environment.

Lack of physical activity is another risk factor for heart disease and stroke by itself but it also leads to obesity and to diabetes, which add to the risk of heart attack and stroke. Obesity increases the strain on the heart, and is directly linked to heart disease because it raises blood pressure, blood cholesterol, and triglyceride levels, and encourages the development of diabetes.

We start getting heavy for a couple of simple reasons. The most important and basic problem is that we take on more calories than we can burn off. While some individuals burn energy more efficiently than others, and thus may find it easier to maintain a healthy weight, everyone can improve weight control by following sound eating habits and getting increased physical activity. It's always a question of balance between calories taken in and the work you do to burn them off.

Reducing the Risks

Knowing the risks of heart disease and stroke is only half the battle. The other half is putting that knowledge to work for the sake of good health and long life. One of the first things you can do is to see your doctor (or find one) and begin a regular schedule of check-ups. Educating yourself is an important step toward reducing heart disease risk. Your doctor will help you begin the education process. Learn your numbers! Know your blood pressure, blood sugar level, and blood cholesterol level (including the good and bad components) and learn where these numbers should normally be for good health.

Then, with your doctor's counsel, stop smoking. Many smoking cessation tools (gum, patches and oral medications) are available to help you safely stop smoking. Your doctor can point you toward support groups that will help you to quit. In addition, health insurance policies will often cover behavior modification programs that can make it easier for you to quit smoking.

You'll have guessed steps three and four. Exercise on a regular basis and eat a healthy diet, with the goal of ending your obesity. Obesity and physical inactivity are two sides of the same coin. Exercise lets you burn off calories and control your weight. Good weight control helps maintain more normal blood pressure, blood sugar, and blood cholesterol.

Food is the fuel for the body, and your body will only be as healthy as the fuel you pump into it. Better food habits can help reduce your risk for heart attack. A healthful eating plan means choosing the right foods to eat and preparing foods in a healthy way. Eat heart smart! And remember, if you watch your weight and keep to a healthy diet you can help prevent or control diabetes, lower high blood pressure and high cholesterol.

Stress

You need to learn how to cope with stress. That's one of the big lifestyle changes you will need to make. It's impossible to keep stress out of our lives, but we can learn how to live with it and not be broken by it. One benefit of exercise is that it provides stress relief.

Besides exercise, another way to reduce stress is through spiritual practice, such as going to church or meditating. Learning to cope with stress is not all easy sliding.

One benefit of exercise is that it provides stress relief.

Often the first step is to get a better grasp of the things that make you tense. In some cases, by managing your life in new ways, you can reduce or eliminate the cause of the stress. But first you must honestly locate it.

For a thorough discussion of stress and stress relief, see *Saving Your Last Nerve,* by Marilyn Martin M.D., M.P.H. (Hilton Publishing, Rockford, IL, 2002).

A more detailed discussion of each risk factor for cardiovascular disease is found in part II of this book. This overview was designed to introduce you to cardiovascular risk factors and to show you how interrelated these risk factors are. That's the reason why one risk modifying strategy (such as exercise), may impact several other risk factors (such as diabetes, blood pressure, or obesity). While there is much to be learned, the rewards of understanding the symptoms of heart disease and the benefit of stress relief for you and your family are great!

CHAPTER 6

HEART DISEASE AND STROKE RISK IN AFRICAN AMERICAN CHILDREN

"Children deserve to know their grandparents so they will become GREAT grandparents." This motto of the Association of Black Cardiologists expresses perfectly the mission of this book—to help you and your family live a long and healthy life.

Our children are our future, and they will carry forward for generations to come our stories, history, culture, arts, and accomplishments. But studies show that heart disease and stroke risk begin in childhood, build up over years, and then cause disabling or fatal heart attacks or strokes in adulthood. Some of these risks are especially likely to be present in African American children and, if untreated, will condemn them to early disability and death.

Women, the caretakers of their families, have the power to change this. Prevention of cardiovascular disease needs to start in childhood so that "children can know their grandparents and become GREAT grandparents themselves."

Studies show that heart disease and stroke risk begin in childhood, build up over years, and then cause disabling or fatal heart attacks or strokes in adulthood. Some of these risks are especially likely to be present in African American children and, if untreated, will condemn them to early disability and death. Women, the caretakers of their families, have the power to change this.

One of the most alarming trends in recent years is the epidemic of cardiovascular risk factors seen in our children. These include:

- Obesity
- Hypertension
- Type 2 diabetes (the kind of diabetes usually seen in middle-aged adults)
- Cigarette smoking

The result of this childhood epidemic of cardiovascular risk factors will be heart attack and stroke, with needless death and disability in early adulthood, unless we take action.

One reason for this deterioration in our childrens' health is that they have become far less physically active. Children no longer walk, jump rope, bicycle, or participate in active play as much as they used to. Recreation is more apt to include watching TV or playing videogames, which are sedentary activities. Physical education in schools is viewed as an "extra" and is often one of the first items to be cut when budgets are tight. After school sports have also dwindled, because safe play areas in cities are lacking. Finally, in families where both parents work, children may not be able to participate in school sports because their parents are not available to drive them to the event or facility. It's not surprising, then, that obesity in children has increased fourfold in the past two decades. The highest rates of obesity are found in African American, Native American and Latino children. Being overweight or obese in childhood and adolescence is associated with:

- Increased risk of hypertension in childhood
- Type 2 diabetes in childhood
- High-risk cholesterol profiles
- Early atherosclerosis.

High blood pressure (hypertension) is one of the most important consequences of obesity, and high blood pressure occurs with greater severity and at earlier ages in African Americans. High blood pressure that begins in childhood and adolescence predicts the development of high blood pressure in adulthood.

Type 2 diabetes (the kind generally seen in middle-aged adults) has increased dramatically in children. Children with Type 2 diabetes are at risk for earlier complications of diabetes, such as blindness, heart disease and kidney disease. The CDC estimates that one in three American children born in the year 2000, will develop diabetes sometime during his or her life.

High blood cholesterol in childhood or adolescence is associated with atherosclerosis later in life. A diet high in saturated fats and cholesterol can increase blood cholesterol levels in the young as well as in adults.

Cigarette smoking is the most serious avoidable health threat. It causes high rates of heart disease, stroke, cancer, and unhealthy pregnancies. Smoking in households also increases childhood respiratory infections, asthma, and childhood deaths. Most smokers begin to smoke in adolescence, and studies show that when smoking begins at young ages it is far more difficult to stop, because nicotine is physically addictive. Smoking is increasingly found (and is more addictive) among young girls than boys. And smoking in young women may be responsible for complicated pregnancies, low-birth-weight infants, and illnesses in children in the household.

How *You* Can Decrease Cardiovascular Risk in Children and Adolescents

For children to live long, healthy lives and become "great grandparents," women need to encourage healthy behaviors and habits in their children to decrease their risk of heart disease and stroke. The big four to be encouraged are:

Physical activity. This should be encouraged by increasing the opportunities for physical play and limiting the number of hours spent watching TV or playing video games. When safety is a consideration, parents should identify safe places for after school play. Encourage children, especially girls, to participate in organized activities, such as sports or dance or just jumping rope. Parents should model a physically active lifestyle by being physically active themselves and encourage active family activities, such as walking, biking, or playing ball as a family. It is important to be involved in your children's school so that you can lobby against curricular changes that might decrease physical education. ***Physical activity is a health issue—not a recreation issue***.

Obesity prevention. This requires more physical activity and less food consumption. It also requires some changes in the kinds of food consumed. A healthy diet is a diet low in saturated fats (fats from animal sources and fried foods) and high in fruits, vegetables, and whole-grain foods. High fat, high carbohydrate junk-food snacks and fast foods (all fried) should be avoided. Substitute fruit and vegetable snacks. Healthy eating habits established in childhood will carry forward into adulthood. After the age of two, children should consume low-fat milk and dairy products. Encourage the whole family to eliminate high carbohydrate, high fat foods and substitute instead whole-grain breads and cereals, fresh fruits and vegetables, baked or broiled meats. Limiting portion size and the number of helpings is also essential.

Extremely overweight children need assistance from health care professionals to reach healthy weights with healthy self-esteem. The American Heart Association recommends the following:

1. Beginning treatment of children before adolescence if possible
2. Having the family participate with the child
3. Educating both family and child about the medical complications of obesity
4. Promoting long-term changes in behavior and diet rather than short term rapid weight loss
5. Emphasizing small and gradual changes
6. Encouragement rather than punishment

Families can work cooperatively to provide the appropriate foods, limit portion size and establish an exercise routine. Team spirit helps everyone on the team.

Prevention of Type 2 diabetes in childhood depends on physical activity and preventing obesity. Children who are at risk (those who are overweight, physically inactive, African American, Native American or Hispanic and who have a family history of diabetes) should be screened for early detection of diabetes. Early diagnosis allows for the most effective treatment. If a child has diabetes, parents or family members must team with health care providers to establish proper nutrition, exercise and medication. Key elements in a family approach to managing childhood diabetes are:

- consume a healthy diet
- limit TV
- exercise together
- drink low-fat milk
- eliminate soda and juices
- eat at home where you can control portion size and fat content.

Be alert to the symptoms of diabetes in your child. These include:

- frequent urination
- excessive thirst
- excessive hunger
- unexplained weight loss
- increased fatigue

- irritability
- changes in vision.

If your child has any of these symptoms seek prompt medical attention.

All children three years old and up should have their blood pressure measured regularly during pediatrician visits. It is particularly important to screen those children at higher risk for hypertension—children who are overweight or who have a family history of hypertension.

Children with hypertension should be seen regularly by their pediatricians, and should follow plans for weight loss, including a

> *It is particularly important to screen those children at higher risk for hypertension.*

reduced salt diet, and increased physical activity instituted with advice from that doctor. Children with persistent or severe hypertension should be evaluated by a specialist, because causes such as kidney disease, blood vessel abnormalities or tumors of the adrenal glands may be responsible.

Prevention of smoking in children has two phases. For infants and young children, the most important strategy is to eliminate tobacco smoke in their environment. Parents and caretakers who smoke expose infants and children to the risk of asthma, respiratory infections, and a behavioral model of "smoking as O.K."

Parents and caretakers of children and young adolescents should discourage experimentation with smoking and emphasize the harmful health consequences of tobacco smoking. That lesson is best taught to your children when your home is smoke-free.

Talk with your children about how they can resist peer-pressure to smoke. It's a key lesson, not only in keeping your children away from smoking but from other threats to their health as well.

Adolescents who smoke may require further assistance from health care providers or community-based programs especially directed to teenagers.

We leave you with this message: because you care about your children, protect their health. It's you, the African American mother, who can best teach them health lessons. Remind them that by following these lessons, they will get to know their grandparents, and live to become loving and helping grandparents themselves. For your children, for yourself, for the community, for the future, act now!

PART II

Heart Disease and Stroke Risk, Prevention, and Management

CHAPTER 7

MANAGING HIGH BLOOD PRESSURE

Hypertension (high blood pressure) is called "the silent killer" for good reason. Women can die of this disease without ever knowing they had it. Among African American women this is especially true. The death rate from high blood pressure is 290% higher for African American women than for their white counterparts.

Hypertension increases the work load on the heart, kidneys, blood vessels, and even the brain. Alone, or along with excess weight, sedentary lifestyle, diabetes, and other risks, hypertension can increase your chances of dying from heart attack and/or stroke.

WHAT IS HIGH BLOOD PRESSURE AND WHY IS IT DANGEROUS?

Blood pressure is the force generated by the heart to pump blood throughout the body. When blood vessels are elastic (compliant) less force is required. When they are stiff, greater force is required to pump blood through them. While this greater force may get blood circulated through stiff, resistant blood vessels, the excess force can eventually damage large and small blood vessels, and in that way damage organs that these blood vessels supply. High blood pressure also requires the heart to work harder and can cause heart enlargement and finally heart failure.

Blood pressure is measured using a two part scale—a top number (measuring systolic pressure) and a bottom number (measuring diastolic pressure). The top number measures the force necessary for blood to be pumped, and the bottom number indicates the force during the time the heart relaxes between beats. A normal blood pressure is less than 120/80 mm Hg. Pre-hypertension is defined as 120–139/80–89. Blood pressure greater than, or equal to, 140/90 mm Hg is called *Stage I Hypertension*, and blood pressure greater than, or equal to, 160/100 mm Hg is *Stage II Hypertension*.

Even if your blood pressure is only moderately elevated, you need to get it back as close as possible to normal (120/80 or lower).

The elevation of either the *top* or *bottom* number indicates high blood pressure, so **140/80** or 130/90 are both defined as unhealthy elevated blood pressures. If either top, bottom, or both numbers are high, they must be reduced.

Recent studies have shown that, even if your blood pressure is only moderately elevated, you need to get it back as close as possible to normal (120/80 or lower).

Remember these slogans: "lower is better" and "every millimeter counts." Even a 3–4 point reduction in blood pressure is important to your health. If you have diabetes, it is especially important to get your blood pressure as close to normal as possible, since hypertension combined with diabetes produces greater damage to blood vessels and organs than either problem alone.

High blood pressure usually has no warning symptoms. Your first symptom may be a stroke, heart attack, sudden death, kidney failure, or damage to other body organs. That's why doctors and patients alike must closely monitor blood pressure. By so doing, you and your doctor help reduce the risk of heart attack, heart failure, stroke, and kidney disease.

The only way you can bring hypertension under control is by following your doctor's orders. It means making lifestyle changes—in particular, getting enough exercise, eating a proper diet, watching your weight, and managing your stress. If lifestyle changes alone fail to control blood pressure, using medications prescribed by your doctor will usually control blood pressure. But, even when medications are used, it is essential to continue to practice a combination of lifestyle changes—exercise, a diet low in salt, high in fruits and vegetables, weight control—and medications to achieve good blood pressure control. Though this may seem daunting at first, good blood pressure control is worth it because it will reduce your risk of heart attack, stroke, kidney failure, and dementia.

Be advised that the changes you must make are not temporary. You *must* continue both the medical treatments and the lifestyle changes all your life if you are to maintain normal blood pressure. But the payoff is worth it: before long, you will feel better and have more energy. Establishing good health habits requires more work than taking medications does, but your own health (and even life) may depend on it.

Following the doctor's order and making it a part of your

daily schedule will not only make you feel good physically, but it will also make you proud. You'll begin to feel like a woman who's in command and control of her own health.

TREATMENT OF HYPERTENSION

Keep in mind that these bad consequences of high blood pressure don't have to happen. Start looking after yourself and your loved ones now, by arranging to get your family's blood pressure checked. For you and any family member with hypertension, the following actions are crucial to blood pressure control:

1. Decrease the salt in your diet
2. Exercise
3. Control weight
4. Stop Smoking
5. Take your medications as prescribed
6. Learn to manage stress

The first components of high blood pressure management are lifestyle modifications. These include:

1. Decrease the salt in your diet. No salt should be added to food. Use spices, herbs, or garlic for flavor. When consuming prepared foods, choose those labeled "low sodium" or "low salt."
2. Begin an exercise program, after getting the okay from your doctor. Exercise should be done at least 30 minutes per day—what exercise you do is less important than the regularity and intensity of that exercise.

Walking briskly, swimming, biking, rowing or dancing are all good choices.

3. Losing weight if you are overweight or obese. A combination of reduced food intake and increased activity will be required to achieve and maintain weight loss.

4. Stopping smoking as quickly as possible.

5. Take your medications if your doctor thinks this is necessary. There are many medications available for the treatment of high blood pressure. While some medications may have undesirable side effects, by trying different combinations of medicines, your healthcare provider should be able to control blood pressure without the side effects. It is important that you take your medicines as directed every day and that you discuss side effects with your doctor. Don't just stop medications assuming all have the same set of side effects. If the cost of these medications is an issue, be very direct about this with your health care provider. Many effective blood pressure medicines are available in generic forms at much lower costs than brand named varieties. Most patients will require more than one agent to control blood pressure.

6. Stress reduction techniques such as meditation, prayer or counseling. These may help you achieve tranquility in your life.

Control of your blood pressure calls for patience and commitment on your part. Lifestyle changes take effort and may not come easily. But the reduction in the risk of heart attack, stroke, kidney failure, and early death is worth the effort.

CHAPTER 8

How *Diabetes Mellitus* Hurts Your Heart

O ne of the most serious risk factors for heart disease and stroke in women is diabetes mellitus (sugar diabetes). *Diabetes mellitus* causes metabolism abnormalities that result in high blood sugar (glucose), and high cholesterol with more bad than good cholesterol. A recent survey in the January/ February issue of the ABC *Digest of Urban Cardiology*, a publication of the Association of Black Cardiologists, revealed a large knowledge gap in the African American community about diabetes and its consequences. Education about diabetes is critical and may save your life.

Diabetes is often accompanied by high blood pressure, further increasing the risk to a woman's heart. Diabetes occurs more commonly in African-Americans and Native Americans than in other ethnic groups. It is the sixth ranked cause of death in the United States, and 75% of deaths in diabetics are caused by cardiovascular disease. People with diabetes are two to four times more likely to have a heart attack or stroke than non-diabetics.

To understand diabetes, think about what happens to food after you swallow it. Nutrients are extracted from that food, and the nutrients are circulated by the blood stream and passed into cells, to be used for energy, or into special organs (fat tissue and the liver) where it can be stored. Insulin, a hormone secreted by the pancreas, helps move nutrients from the bloodstream into your cells where it may be used for energy or stored for later use.

Diabetes results from two kinds of abnormalities.

Type I diabetes occurs when there is complete failure of the pancreas to secrete insulin so nutrients cannot move into cells and blood sugar is very high. This type of diabetes is the most common type of diabetes in childhood, but it makes up only 10% of all cases.

Type II diabetes ("maturity onset diabetes") is the most common type of diabetes in adults, and has a mixture of causes. Early in the course of the disease the body secretes enough, or even more than enough, insulin, but the cells that would normally respond to it become less sensitive to the effects of insulin (insulin resistance), and so glucose (sugar) in the blood is not moved into cells for either energy or storage. Insulin resistance is often accompanied by high blood pressure, obesity and unfavorable cholesterol levels.

The liver, which normally stores and releases glucose between meals, may release glucose inappropriately, further increasing the level of glucose in the blood. Finally, with time, the pancreas wears out and fails to produce insulin. The result of all these processes is high blood glucose. Levels of cholesterol and blood fats called triglycerides are also abnormally high and contribute to damage to both large and small blood vessels.

Complications of Diabetes

Regardless of the type of diabetes, the long-standing elevation in blood sugar, cholesterol and triglycerides is extremely harmful to the cardiovascular system. The very smallest blood vessels in the kidney may be damaged, leading to kidney failure and the need to be on dialysis. When diabetes coexists with hypertension, the damage to the kidney is much greater than from each condition alone. When the smallest blood vessels in the eyes are affected, blindness may result.

Diabetes may also damage the nerves to the legs and hands, resulting in numbness, tingling, and painful sensations that are difficult to treat. Diabetes frequently damages the blood vessels to the legs and feet so that these extremities don't receive an adequate supply of blood and nutrients. Because of this, a minor injury to the leg or foot can't heal. These small, injured areas can become infected, sometimes requiring amputation of the limb.

A particularly important complication of diabetes is that it speeds up the development of cholesterol plaque in the arteries of the heart and brain, thus increasing the risk for heart attacks and strokes.

An important kind of diabetes for women is diabetes that occurs during pregnancy and clears up, or resolves after delivery. It occurs in 2–5 % of pregnancies overall but in up to 14% in certain ethnic groups. Untreated diabetes in pregnancy can result in high maternal and infant death, as well as in other complications of pregnancy.

Screening for diabetes in pregnancy should be done for all women, but particularly in women

- Who are obese

- Have a strong family history of diabetes
- Are African American or other ethnic group, such as Native American, where the prevalence of diabetes is high,
- Have delivered a baby greater than nine pounds (diabetic women commonly have large babies, but these babies may not be as healthy as babies born to non-diabetic women)
- Have had prior diabetes with pregnancy.

All women over 45 years of age should be screened, as should those under 45 if they:

- Are obese or overweight
- Have a family history of diabetes (particularly parents or siblings)
- Belong to a high risk ethnic group (African-American, Native American, Hispanic-American, Asian-Pacific Islander)
- Have high blood pressure
- Have had diabetes with pregnancy

SYMPTOMS OF DIABETES

Women with diabetes often experience excessive hunger, excessive thirst, weight loss, and frequent urination. They may also feel unusual fatigue, and in some, cases lethargy and sleepiness. When diabetes goes untreated for a prolonged time and blood sugars are very high, coma and death may result.

Management of Diabetes

Management of diabetes requires a close working relationship with a health-care team expert in the treatment of this disease. These professionals should include a physician, nurse/educator, nutritionist, and exercise specialist.

The goal of treatment is to maintain the patient's blood sugar as close as possible to normal, and to prevent long term complications of diabetes, such as kidney failure, blindness, nerve damage, heart attack and stroke. The cornerstones of care are:

1. *Daily Blood sugar monitoring*—essential so that diet, exercise and medication can be adjusted accordingly. In addition, as a measurement of long-term control of blood sugar, the Hemoglobin A_1C test should be done quarterly.

2. *Nutritional guidelines* should be worked out with a dietician and scrupulously followed. Nutritional guidelines need to be individualized to take into consideration the patient's lifestyle, exercise habits, eating preferences, and culture.

3. *Weight management* is extremely important because obesity increases insulin resistance. Some people are able to manage diabetes just by weight loss, diet and exercise without the help of medication. Alternatively, lower doses of medications may be necessary if weight loss is successful.

4. *Exercise* is also a specific therapy for diabetes. Exercise helps your body to be more sensitive to insulin so less is required, and exercise also helps you to maintain

leaner body weight. An exercise plan should be worked out with your health care provider.

5. *Medications* are also used There are several kinds of medicine for diabetes that can be taken by mouth. Another medication, insulin, must be taken as a daily injection. Your health care provider will determine which is the best combination of medications for you and work with you to achieve good control of blood sugars.

PREVENTIVE CARE

Because of the complications of diabetes, it is critical that diabetic patients have the following preventive care:

- Regular blood pressure checks
- Quarterly measurement of A_1C
- Regular tests of kidney function
- Regular eye exams by an eye specialist
- Regular tests of cholesterol and triglycerides
- Good care of the feet to prevent sores that may not heal

Diabetes is a chronic (long-term) disease that has to be managed by patients in a good working relationship with a multidisciplinary health care team. The best way to approach this disease is first to know whether you are at risk for it, then to be regularly screened, and then, if diabetes is identified, to work with your healthcare team to modify diet, reduce weight, exercise, and take medications as prescribed.

CHAPTER 9

CHOLESTEROL AND YOUR BLOOD VESSELS

Cholesterol has become a household word—everyone knows it's bad for your health if there is too much in your bloodstream and that Americans, in general, have too much cholesterol. This issue, however, is a bit more complicated than that.

Cholesterol is one kind of lipid (fatty substance) found in the bloodstream. It gets into the bloodstream in two ways. First, the body manufactures cholesterol because it's necessary. Cholesterol makes up a part of the walls of individual cells. Second, cholesterol may also be absorbed from foods we eat that contain the substance (such as eggs and shrimp) or made by the body from saturated fats (such as bacon and animal fats) in the diet.

Hyperlipidemia is the name given to an excess of lipid (fat) molecules in the bloodstream. There are several kinds of lipids, or fats, which when excessive, can damage blood vessels. Hypercholesterolemia (high cholesterol) is one form of hyperlipidemia. It is the form most hazardous to your cardiovascular health. When too much cholesterol is present in the blood-stream, plaques, which block blood flow, are more likely to develop within the vessel walls. Other damaging events occur at the site of a plaque and include the overgrowth of certain cell types and the migration of inflammatory cells and clot forming cells to the site. Blood vessels with such plaques may also have abnormal spasm at those sites, resulting in further decreases of blood flow to the heart and other organs.

At some point, the inflammation at the site of a plaque increases to a level that causes the breakdown or rupture of the overlying vessel lining. When that happens, a clot forms at the site of the rupture. The clot can completely block the artery, leading to a heart attack or stroke. And thus, excess cholesterol, over a period of years, can increase the risk of heart attack.

It is important to understand that there are several kinds of cholesterol which should be measured.

- *Total cholesterol* is the sum of all the different kinds of cholesterol in the body.
- *LDL cholesterol* is the bad cholesterol. When elevated in the bloodstream, LDL cholesterol will move out of the blood and be deposited into the blood vessel walls. LDL cholesterol is the main source of irritation and inflamma-tion in the vessel wall and it is the kind of cholesterol that leads to formation of plaque in the vessel wall.
- *HDL cholesterol* is the good cholesterol. It serves as a "vacuum cleaner," cleaning up the LDL cholesterol, and removing it from the system so it can't be deposited within the vessel wall. The most favorable cholesterol

situation is to have a *low total cholesterol,* a *low LDL cho-lesterol* and a *high HDL cholesterol.* The following table will provide the cholesterol numbers that are considered best for you. The reason it's important to have all three cholesterol components measured is that when LDL cho-lesterol is elevated and /or HDL cholesterol is low, risk of heart attack is increased, even if the total cholesterol level is within normal limits.

More recently, *triglycerides* (another fatty substance in the blood derived from food intake) have also been shown to have an association with the increased risk of developing plaques leading to heart attack and stroke. Triglycerides may also be elevated when diabetes is poorly controlled, thus adding to the heart risk of diabetes. In general, a complete lipid profile will include meas-uring the total cholesterol, LDL and HDL cholesterols, and the triglyceride level. Table 1 shows the optimal levels.

The National Cholesterol Education Program (NCEP) has devised guidelines for treatment of cholesterol called the Adult Treatment Panel. This 2001 report represents a major update of previous guidelines. The new guidelines call for more aggressive

---

Table 1. **Optimal Cholesterol and Triglyceride Levels**

TC less than 200
LDL less than 100 optimal
HDL greater than 40 (greater than 50 in women) optimal
Triglyceride less than 150 optimal

diagnosis and treatment of hypercholesterolemia, especially when associated with coronary artery disease or with risk factors for coronary disease (such as diabetes, hypertension). Table 1 shows what is now considered a normal LDL and HDL cholesterol level and what is considered the upper limits of normal for triglyceride level. When you have a cholesterol test done, be sure that the different kinds of cholesterol and triglycerides are measured in addition to the total cholesterol. This is important because an individual may have a total cholesterol level of less than 200 but have a high LDL level, which would place that person in a high risk category. On the other hand, the same total cholesterol level with low LDL and high HDL levels would place the individual at low risk for cardiovascular disease. Ask your healthcare providers to test all of your cholesterol numbers and to discuss them with you.

Treatment of hyperlipidemia revolves around diet, behavior modification (called "therapeutic lifestyle change" in the NCEP guidelines), and medical therapy. Therapeutic lifestyle change incorporates a diet of reduced saturated fats (those fats derived from animal sources or those that are solid at room temperature), high levels of fruit, vegetables, and fiber and cholesterol intake of less than 200 mg/day. Therapeutic lifestyle change also incorporates weight reduction programs and increased regular physical exercise.

When cholesterol cannot be lowered to normal, healthy levels, medication may be necessary. There are several different types of medications to lower cholesterol on the market now. Over the past twenty years, multiple studies have conclusively shown a decrease in death and heart attack when medications are used for treatment of high levels of cholesterol. This result has been shown in groups with severe, moderate, and even low risk. If your doctor recommends a medicine to control cholesterol, be assured that your risk of heart disease, in all likelihood, will be reduced. These medicines work in several ways—some decrease the production of cholesterol by the body, some prevent dietary cholesterol from being absorbed from food by either binding to cholesterol in the intestine or preventing it from crossing the intestinal wall and entering the bloodstream. Your healthcare provider will determine which medication is most appropriate and will do periodic blood tests to be sure your cholesterol is at the right level.

The most important thing you can do for yourself is to have your cholesterol checked. When you do, make sure you have the total cholesterol, LDL, HDL, and triglycerides measured. If these don't meet the optimal levels in Table 1, you and your healthcare provider can initiate a treatment plan that includes diet, exercise, weight reduction and, possibly, medications to bring these values into the appropriate range. Your treatment program should be tailored to reach your cholesterol goals with the least amount of side effects.

CHAPTER 10

TOBACCO AND YOUR HEART

THE BAD NEWS

Tobacco smoking is responsible for more than 400,000 deaths each year, or 1 in 5 deaths, making tobacco smoking the single greatest cause of premature death and disease in America today. Half of all regular smokers die prematurely of a tobacco-related illness. Eighty percent of those people who smoke cigarettes begin before age 18, with the most common age of initiation being 14–15. Among African American females over the age of 18, one in five consider themselves to be smokers.

About 35,000 *nonsmokers* will die from coronary heart disease each year as a result of exposure to tobacco smoke in the environment. Children exposed to environmental smoke have a high prevalence of asthma (which can be fatal) and respiratory infections. Smoking costs Americans over $257 billion annually in medical care. These large human costs are devastating and can be avoided. You cannot live in the twentieth century and not know about the high medical risk of tobacco smoke. Smoking increases the:

- Risk of heart attack, and stroke
- Risk of lung disease and emphysema
- Risk of several cancers, including lung cancer, head and neck cancer, and bladder cancer.

Young women may start smoking during the teen years as a way to appear cool and glamorous. Rest assured that people with cancer of the head and neck who have had portions of their jaws and faces removed do not feel so cool or glamorous. Dying from lung cancer, emphysema, heart attack or stroke is not a glamorous way to die.

How does smoking affect the heart and blood vessels? Within minutes of inhaling tobacco smoke, blood vessels respond by constricting, or narrowing, so that the blood supply to essential organs is reduced.

Smoking on a regular basis damages the lining of the blood vessels leading to cholesterol build-up and plaque development. All of the blood vessels in the body are damaged, leading to widespread development of atherosclerotic (cholesterol) plaques. As a result, smokers develop poor circulation to the heart, brain and limbs, leading to heart attack, strokes and amputation of limbs.

When smoking is combined with other risk factors, such as physical inactivity, hypertension, diabetes, or hypercholesterolemia, the harm to the body increases dramatically. Women who have more than two risk factors and smoke are at especially high risk for heart disease and stroke at an early age. Young women who smoke and use birth control pills are also at very high risk of heart attack and stroke at ages as young as the teens and twenties.

The Good News . . .

Since 1965, smoking has declined over 40% among people age 18 and older in the United States. From 1980 to 2001, the percentage of high school seniors who smoked in the past month decreased almost 50% in the African American population. So we are doing something right, but much more needs to be done.

Community education has helped and the anti-smoking campaign has won significant victories. As a result of lawsuits directed against tobacco companies, the tobacco companies were court-ordered to spend money on public service announcements that tell the truth about the health consequences of tobacco use. Do-not-smoke campaigns were given new life in the United States.

Treatment

A smoker has to want to quit to stand a chance at long-term success. People who are quitting will experience a range of behavioral and physical withdrawal symptoms following smoking cessation, including irritability, anger, impatience, restlessness, and more. It is important for women to understand that their withdrawal symptoms may be much more severe than those of men, because nicotine has stronger effects on women.

Even with the best treatment, only about 1 in 3 smokers remains off tobacco one year after they've "stopped". Smokers

---

Table 1. **Physical symptoms of nicotine withdrawal**

Irritability

Anger

Impatience

Restlessness

Difficulty concentrating

Insomnia

Increased appetite

Anxiety

Depressed mood

Agency for Health Care Policy and Research (AHCPR) 1996 (www.surgeon-general.gov/tobacco)

---

with depression have a more difficult time quitting, but many *do* succeed.

Smoking is a completely learned experience. That's why behaviors and cues normally associated with smoking or, "lighting up," must be unlearned. For instance,

- Smokers frequently have a cigarette with a drink or after a meal.
- Smokers frequently smoke to relieve stress.
- Eventually, cigarettes can become a way to keep your hands busy.
- Smokers often become accustomed to placing something in their mouths.

Table 2A. **Five Common Myths About Quitting Smoking**

Myth 1   Smoking is just a bad habit.

Myth 2   Quitting is just a matter of willpower.

Myth 3   If you can't quit the first time you try, you will never be able to quit.

Myth 4   The best way to quit is "cold turkey."

Myth 5   Quitting is expensive.

Table 2B. **The Truth About Quitting Smoking**

Fact 1   Tobacco use is an addiction, as addictive as heroin or cocaine for some people. The addiction potential of cigarettes is higher for women than men.

Fact 2   Because smoking is an addiction, quitting is often very difficult. A number of treatments are available that can help.

Fact 3   Quitting is hard. Usually people try two or three times or more before being able to quit for good.

Fact 4   The most effective way to quit smoking is by using a combination of counseling, behavioral approaches and nicotine replacement therapy or non-nicotine medica-tion. Your health care provider or smoking cessation clinic is the best place to go for help with quitting.

Fact 5   Treatments cost from $3 to $10 dollars per day. A pack-a-day smoker spends almost $1000 per year. Check with your health insurance plan to find out if smoking ces-sation medications and /or counseling are covered.

*Agency for Health Care Policy and Research (AHCPR) 1996 (*www.surgeon-general.gov/tobacco)

Table 3. **Good Reasons for Quitting**

- Over 400,000 Americans die each year from smoking
- When you quit, your chances of getting sick from smoking will be less
- When you quit, you will have more energy and breathe easier
- If you are pregnant, your baby will get more oxygen and be healthier
- The people you live with, especially your children, will be healthier. Breathing in other people's smoke can cause asthma and other health problems in children.

Agency for Health Care Policy and Research (AHCPR) 1996 (www.surgeon-general.gov/tobacco)

These cues, or behaviors, must be unlearned in order to achieve long-term successful smoking cessation.

While the chief obstacle to quitting smoking is the addictive nature of nicotine, to ensure success, treatment must use a combined approach. While the patient must do a good part of the work, simply by deciding firmly that he or she wants to quit, there are also medications that help relieve the symptoms of tobacco withdrawal. Nicotine patches, gums, vapors, or inhalers (as needed) along with oral non-nicotine medications, have all been shown to work well, particularly in the smoker with associated depression.

The most studied non-nicotine medication is *bupropion*. This medication was initially used as an antidepressant, and is still occasionally used in this role. However, it is also quite successful in helping individuals to stop smoking.

There is some controversy over whether combination therapy, (non-nicotine medication together with nicotine medication), is better than non-nicotine medication alone. You should work with your healthcare provider to determine the best medications to assist you.

Counseling and education are also key components to this combined approach. Exercise, too, plays a supporting role, both by maintaining physical fitness and by preventing the 5–10 pound weight gain seen in up to 30% of smokers (especially women) who succeed in quitting. Finally, social support and behavior modification can prevent relapse. By helping smokers to learn new cues and behaviors, as well as to avoid the old ones and the people connected with them—quitting tobacco use is quite achievable.

The combined approach has the highest rate of success. Even brief interventions by your physician during an office visit can help you to stop smoking. Tables 4 and 5 outline a strategy to stop smoking designed by the Department of Health and Human Services.

Preparing to stop on a specific date requires a little planning. Table 4 gives you some suggestions.

Now that you have set a quit date, Table 5 gives you some ideas about what you can do to stick to your decision to stop smoking.

Table 4. **Five-Day Countdown to Your Quit Date**

Day 5	Think about your reasons for quitting. Tell your friends and family you are planning to quit. Stop buying cigarettes.
Day 4	Pay attention to when and why you smoke. Think of other things to hold in your hand instead of a cigarette. Think of habits or routines to change.
Day 3	What will you do with the extra money when you stop buying cigarettes? Think of whom to reach out to when you need help.
Day 2	Buy the nicotine patch or nicotine gum. Or see your doctor to get the nicotine inhaler, nasal spray, or the non-nicotine pill.
Day 1	Put away lighters and ashtrays. Throw away all cigarettes and matches. Clean your clothes to get rid of the smell of cigarette smoke.
Quit Day	Keep very busy. Remind family and friends that this is your quit day. Stay away from alcohol. Give yourself a treat, or do something special. If you "slip" and smoke, don't give up. Set a new date to get back on track. Call a friend or "quit smoking" support group. Eat healthy food and get exercise.

*Agency for Health Care Policy and Research (AHCPR) 1996 (*www.surgeon-general.gov/tobacco)

Table 5. **Strategy for Smoking Cessation**

- Change the things around you (get rid of all cigarettes and ashtrays at home, in your car, and at your place of work).
- After you quit, don't smoke, not even a puff!
- Ask your pharmacist about the nicotine patch or gum, which can be bought at a drugstore
- Ask your doctor about other prescription medications, such as bupropion, a nicotine inhaler, or nicotine nasal spray.
- Ask your family, friends, and people you work with for their support.
- Get together with other people who are trying to quit. To find out where to get help in your area, call the American Cancer Society (1–800–ACS–2345).
- If you slip, don't give up. Set a new quit date and get back on track.
- Avoid alcohol.
- Avoid being around others who are smoking
- Eat healthy food and get exercise.
- Keep a positive attitude!

Most people try to quit several times before they quit for good. Quitting is hard, but you CAN DO IT! Remember, there has never been a better time to quit!

*Agency for Health Care Policy and Research (AHCPR) 1996 (*www.surgeon-general.gov/tobacco)

CHAPTER 11

OBESITY, EXERCISE AND DIET
The Scope of the Problem

Obesity and becoming overweight has become an American healthcare epidemic. Fully ninety-seven million Americans are obese, which is defined as being 30% or more over one's ideal body weight.

The prevalence of being overweight and obese is much higher in African American women compared to the rest of the population, with some 37% of African American women being obese.

These alarmingly high rates of obesity can be translated into increased health costs, poorer health in general, higher rates of heart disease, diabetes, high blood pressure, some cancers and an increased death rate. The total health-care costs due to obesity were $99.2 billion in 1995. $51.6 billion dollars were medical costs directly associated with obesity; $47.6 billion were indirect costs representing the value of lost work caused by illness and death. For people who meet the definition of being obese (221 pounds with a height of 6' 0" and 186 pounds at a height of

5'6"), death from all causes, especially from cardiovascular causes, increased by 50–100% above that of people of normal weight.

Obesity, in and of itself, is considered a risk factor for heart disease. The problem, however, is that obesity is almost always found with other risk factors for heart disease, such as hypertension, diabetes, hyperlipidemia, and smoking. When this happens, the risk of heart disease is even greater.

Weight reduction can improve cardiovascular risk in the following ways: It helps to reduce blood pressure, improve blood sugars for those who are diabetic, and results in reduced cholesterol and triglyceride levels. In addition, weight reduction can help prevent diseases from developing. For those with a family history of diabetes, maintenance of normal body weight and exercise may prevent or delay the development of diabetes.

For smokers who are obese, there is an additional challenge. When you stop smoking the health benefits can be profound: You'll decrease the risk of cancer, heart attack and stroke. However, you may gain weight after you stop smoking. Because trying to stop smoking is difficult and stressful, doctors often tell patients to stop smoking first, then reduce weight; but don't try to do both at the same time. Taking these actions one at a time will improve your chances of success for both.

Diagnosis

Being overweight is defined as being 10% over your ideal body weight; being obese is defined as being 30% over your ideal body weight. Ideal body weight has traditionally been determined from life insurance tables created by Mutual Life Insurance Company of New York. These tables were developed in the

1960s and based on ethnically homogenous populations. In addition, height is not accounted for. A person 6 feet tall will carry 180 pounds better than a person 5' 2" tall. Therefore, the insurance definition of "ideal" has more recently been replaced by the concept of *body mass index* or BMI. Body mass index is expressed in weight in kilograms, rather than pounds adjusted, for height. Height is expressed in meters, not feet. Therefore, body mass index is expressed in units of kg/m^2. To determine BMI when weight is measured in pounds and height in feet, a formula is used to convert these units.

Determining BMI

BMI = (kg/m^2).

To determine your BMI: weight in lbs/2.2 ÷ height in inches x .0254

The numbers 2.2 and 0.0254 are to convert pounds and inches to kilograms and $meters^2$.

Normal BMI is equal to 20—25 kg/m^2

Overweight BMI is equal to 25—29.9 kg/m^2

Obese BMI is equal to, or greater than, 30 kg/m^2

Extreme Obesity is equal to, or greater than, 40 kg/m^2

The reason to take an individual's height into account when considering weight is because cardiovascular risk appears to be more closely linked to the combination of height and weight rather than to weight alone. Using the BMI index, being overweight is defined as having a BMI of between 25–29.9 kg/m². Obesity is defined as having a BMI 30 kg/m² or greater.

Being overweight and being obese can also be determined by measuring your waist (that is, taking the size of your waist). The reason this measurement is useful is that the presence of excess fat in the abdomen—which shows up as a higher waist measurement—increases a person's risk of developing other conditions such as hypertension, hyperlipidemia, diabetes, and heart disease. The Department of Health and Human Services has devised a specific way to measure waist circumference. To define the level at which waist circumference is measured, a bony landmark is first located and marked. The patient stands and the examiner, positioned to the right of the subject, feels for the upper hip bone to locate the tip of the pelvis on the right side. A horizontal mark is drawn. The plane of the tape must be parallel to the floor and the tape must be snug, but should not compress the skin. The waist circumference is measured at this position with normal breathing. *A waist measurement of 35 or more inches indicates obesity.*

Waist circumference measurements are not as accurate above a BMI of 35 kg/ m², but can give some estimate of the degree to which a person is overweight.

When used together, measuring BMI and taking your waist measurement are powerful indicators of a person's risk of heart-related problems, compared to a person of normal weight (see the following table) and can help in making a decision about whether a weight reduction program is needed.

What is your Body Mass Index? _____

What is your waist measurement? _____

Treatment

Treating obesity normally centers around reducing and managing weight. Weight control contributes to the control of cardiovascular risk factors, such as hypertension, diabetes, and high cholesterol. Treatment of obesity, therefore, should focus on producing substantial weight loss over a long period of time and include:

- behavior modification to reduce food intake
- low calorie diets
- exercise and increased physical activity generally
- medications and/or surgery in selected cases.

Keep in mind that weight loss is a process requiring a combined approach of *decreased* energy (food) intake and *increased* energy expenditure. It also requires commitment to a permanent change in diet and exercise in order to maintain weight loss. Therefore, a weight management program should be put into place once weight loss is achieved. Weight management programs should consist of the following:

- regular exercise program
- long-term nutritional guidance
- behavior modification to avoid potentially destructive eating behavior

- education in stress reduction techniques.
- social support

A good support system can provide immense emotional strength to you during weight loss and weight management phases. Some people benefit from formal weight loss and weight management programs sponsored by fitness clubs, YMCAs or YWCAs, and weight loss programs such as Weight Watchers®, NutriSystems®, or Jenny Craig®. However, a church health group, or just a group of committed friends, can provide the same support.

For those with extreme obesity, there are many weight loss medications now on the market. Each, however, has its own benefits and side effects and must be discussed thoroughly with your doctor before you begin to take any of them. Keep in mind also that lifestyle changes in diet and exercise will still be necessary to maintain weight loss.

Weight loss medications should be saved for those people with a BMI over 40, or 35–39.9 if they have conditions that increase their risk of developing cardiovascular disease. For extreme obesity, there are also surgical therapies available. Presently, the most popular surgeries for weight reduction are stomach bypass or stomach reduction surgery. Surgery will not cure obesity but will help an individual reduce weight by restricting the amount of food that person can ingest. However, a combination of interventions is almost always necessary to maintain weight loss. The individual going through the surgery must have strong social support, receive continuous, long-term nutritional guidance, and put in place a long-term exercise program. Surgery, to be successful, means a life-long lifestyle change.

Exercise

What's important in exercise is less *what* exercise you do than how regularly you do it. The health benefits of regular exercise have been demonstrated in many populations and cultures. It doesn't matter what exercise you pick, as long as you find something you enjoy and can do regularly. People exercise in a variety of ways. The simplest, and perhaps the most common form of good exercise is just plain walking. Others will choose bicycling, swimming, dancing, or aerobics.

The benefits of regular exercise:

- Reduced blood pressure
- Reduced risk of diabetes
- Better control of diabetes if a woman already has the condition
- Weight reduction, if desired, or, if you're already at the right weight, a means of staying there
- Prevention of age-related bone thinning (osteoporosis) in women
- Reduced rates of some cancers

You should consult a physician before beginning an exercise program. Your doctor or health-care provider can tell you what regimen is healthy for you and what is not, and she can point you to groups or programs that will help you get going and keep going. If you've chosen walking as your exercise but don't feel safe walking alone in your neighborhood, walk with a group of women, or at a public place such as a mall. Join or form a church group committed to regular exercise.

You may also want to consider joining the YWCA or YMCA (both organizations are co-ed.) If cost is a concern, ask your Y manager for an application for an adjusted fee. The forms are simple, and all Ys have programs allowing you to pay according to your income, or sometimes for no fee at all.

If you haven't exercised for a long time this may be hard to believe, but for most people who get into regular exercise schedules, exercise is fun. You'll begin to notice changes in your stamina and your sense of well-being. You may sleep better and have less of an appetite. You'll also find, if you're like most of the people who exercise regularly, that you get sick less often and have less trouble with stress and depression. Exercise is a natural mood elevator. Exercise gives you an opportunity to concentrate your mind on your body. That means you can turn off your thoughts for a while and in that way get a little time off from the stress you brought in with you. That "time off," if you keep to your routine, eventually becomes part of your everyday life. Exercise is very much like meditation

Exercise also gives you a chance to set yourself little goals and meet them. In that way, you will feel more confident when you face larger goals. Exercise is a great teacher of will power.

These benefits can come so easily, if you want them. Let's say you decide to work out in a gym. Maybe you want to use weights, but can't manage anything heavier than a five-pound weight. Start there. Keep at it for a couple of weeks, at least three times a week. Soon, the five-pound weights will feel too light, and the ten-pound weights will feel just right. And so on.

For exercise to work, it must be regular. Whatever exercise you choose, do it at least three times a week, then advance to the point where you exercise at least thirty minutes each day. It's best to schedule each session at the same time if possible. Another way to increase your energy expenditure is to make opportunities to exercise during ordinary daily activities—take stairs instead of the elevator, park at the far end of the parking lot, rake leaves instead of using a blower, if you have to sit at a desk at work, do leg lifts and arm lifts at regular intervals.

The most important thing about exercise is not *what* you do, but *that you do it* at least thirty minutes per day.

Once you have established a routine, you will be on the road to health, well-being and a longer life.

DIET

In planning heart-healthy dietary patterns, you need to take into consideration factors such as whether or not you have diabetes, high blood pressure, high cholesterol, as well as your weight relative to height. It is therefore important to work with your health care provider and a nutritionist to be sure your diet is tailored to suit your individual needs. The general dietary guidelines for a heart-healthy diet are:

1. Reduce saturated fat intake. Saturated fats are those fats that are derived from animal sources, including beef, lamb, pork, and poultry with the skin on. Whole milk products, butter, cheese, and lard are all high in saturated fats. Some plant-derived oils are also high in saturated fats, including palm and coconut oils and cocoa butter. Foods high in cholesterol, such as eggs, shellfish, liver, brain, and kidney, should be consumed in moderate amounts. The principal dietary driver of

high cholesterol is saturated fats so limiting them in your diet is the healthiest strategy. Substitute unsaturated fats for cooking and for salad dressings. Unsaturated fats include safflower, corn, soybean, sunflower, olive, canola, and peanut oils. While these fats are heart-healthier than saturated fats, they contain the same number of calories as saturated fats and so may contribute to weight gain. The recommendations for the amount of fat in the diet are: less than 10% of the day's calories from *saturated* fats, less than 30% of the day's total calories from any fat, and less than 300 mg of dietary cholesterol per day. Ocean fish such as salmon and mackerel contain a beneficial kind of oil (called omega 3 fatty acids) that is heart-healthy and so should be consumed instead of meat.

2. Increase the amounts of fresh or frozen vegetables in your diet. Vegetables are naturally low in total, as well as saturated, fats, have no cholesterol and are high in fiber. Fiber in the diet lowers cholesterol and slows the absorption of sugars. Fruits and vegetables are also high in vitamins and anti-oxidants, which promote heart-healthiness. Nuts are also excellent for the heart and contain both fiber and selenium, an essential mineral. Nuts are also high in fat so need to be consumed in moderation.

3. Limit sweets, fruit juices and refined carbohydrates, particularly prepared baked goods that are high in sugar and saturated fats. Choose whole-grain bread products rather than white bread products.

4. Limit salt intake. Choose herbs and spices to flavor foods. Seasonings such as onion, garlic, ginger, peppers and lemon juice may be substituted. Avoid using prepared foods, as salt content cannot be controlled. If you do use prepared foods, choose those labeled low sodium or low salt.

The 2000 USDA/USDHHS guidelines for a healthy diet are summarized below:

1. Vegetables—3–5 servings per day
2. Fruits—2–4 servings per day
3. Dairy products—2–3 servings per day
   (skim or 1% fat)
4. Meat, fish, dry beans, eggs, nuts, seeds—2–3 servings per day
   (6 oz lean meat or fish per day)
5. Fats, oils, sweets—use sparingly
6. Breads, cereals, grains—6–11 servings per day

The National Institutes of Health National Heart, Lung, and Blood Institute (NIH/NHLBI) publication *Heart Healthy Handbook for Women* has a set of seven Dietary Guidelines for Americans that are easy to remember and will help you shift to a healthier eating pattern for yourself and your family. These include:

1. Eat a variety of foods
2. Balance what you eat with physical activity

3. Choose a diet with plenty of grains, fruits and vegetables
4. Choose a diet low in total fat, saturated fat and cholesterol
5. Choose a diet moderate in sugars
6. Choose a diet moderate in salt and sodium
7. If you consume alcohol, do so in moderation—for women, no more than one alcoholic beverage per day.

When choosing snacks for you and your family, choose fruits and raw vegetables, unsweetened cereals, baked chips and low-fat dairy treats.

A word or two about vitamin supplements is in order to complete this section. While foods rich in vitamins C, E, and beta-carotene have been shown to be good for you, it is not yet clear that taking these vitamins as supplements is beneficial to health. While it is probably okay to take a multi-vitamin pill per day, research has not proven that anti-oxidant vitamin supplements provide benefits. Therefore, the current recommendation is to consume a diet rich in vitamins and minerals rather than take vitamin supplements.

Making dietary changes requires thought and a bit of work to find ways to prepare tasteful foods low in fat, salt and sugar. It takes about six weeks to change a taste preference or habit, so stick to the new food even if it's difficult at first. Once you get the hang of it, you will find you (and your family's) "taste buds" will shift to healthier choices.

CHAPTER 12

MENOPAUSE

A Woman's Special Cardiovascular Risk

Sometime in middle age, when women come to the end of their capacity to bear children, menopause, or "change of life," occurs. For some women, menopause is an exhilarating time of liberation. It offers freedom from further pregnancies, freedom from having to look "just so," self-assurance, and the wisdom that comes from years of living. For others, menopause is a time of loss: loss of the ability to have babies, loss of youth and the romantic promises of love, as well as loss of that time when there is "more of life ahead than behind." Regardless of which emotional response you experience, the time of menopause also has certain implications for your health, implications that all women need to know.

WHAT IS MENOPAUSE?

Menopause is a normal part of the aging process. In most women, it happens at or around fifty, but it can occur as early as the forties and as late as the mid-fifties. Women who have surgical removal of the ovaries at any age undergo menopause at that time.

Here's how menopause works. When a woman is born, her ovaries contain a certain number of eggs. During adolescence, the onset of menstruation marks the beginning of a monthly cycle. Eggs ripen for fertilization, and if they are fertilized the result is pregnancy. If pregnancy doesn't occur, the eggs are shed with menstrual blood flow. This monthly cycle is controlled by cyclic changes in female hormone levels controlled by the pituitary gland, located in the brain.

Menopause occurs when production of female hormones decreases and the ovaries stop producing eggs in this monthly cycle. The process is gradual, and may extend over an 8–10 year period. During this time, female hormone levels gradually decrease, fertility decreases, and a number of other changes in a woman's body occur, such as weight gain and changes in the places where body fat accumulates. When menstrual periods have been absent for 12 months, the passage through menopause is complete.

While menopause is a normal event, symptoms associated with it may be bothersome. Most women will experience some of these symptoms, but few will have symptoms severe enough to be serious threats to health. The symptoms of menopause are:

- Hot flashes
- Insomnia
- Mood changes
- Mild forgetfulness
- Decreased libido (sexual drive)

- Vaginal dryness
- Thinning of scalp hair
- Urinary flow disturbances.

While these symptoms may be bothersome and distressing, at most they last for a few years. You can relieve the symptoms of menopause by making changes in your lifestyle, including:

- Getting more exercise
- Avoiding spicy foods and alcohol
- Avoiding foods containing nitrites or sulfites (preservatives in foods)
- Adding soy products to your diet.

Short-term hormone replacement therapy will relieve almost all of these symptoms, but it also has some potentially serious risks. (You'll find more on hormone therapy later in this chapter.)

Menopause is a normal part of aging, but it's also a time when risks for certain health problems increase. Thus, while women have lower incidences than men of cardiovascular diseases before menopause, women's risk of cardiovascular diseases increases sharply after menopause. This means that by the seventh and eighth decades of life, women's risk of cardiovascular disease is almost equal to men's.

The risk of osteoporosis (brittle bones) increases at this time also. Everyone knows that female hormones are the substances that cause women to develop female bodies. What may be less well known is that female hormones also affect other kinds of body structures. They help make bones strong and blood vessels flexible and compliant. They also decrease the amount of choles-terol build-up in blood vessels. Thus, in addition to other age-related risk factors (increased high blood pressure, increased cho-lesterol levels, increased incidence of diabetes), loss of estrogen at menopause may contribute to the increased risk of heart disease.

In studies over the past thirty years, researchers noticed that women appeared to be protected from cardiovascular disease before menopause and that female hormones taken after menopause appeared to protect the blood vessels from choles-terol build-up. It seemed reasonable that treating women with hormones after menopause might be helpful. In studies where women who chose to take hormones after menopause were com-pared to women who chose not to, the hormone users appeared to have lower incidences of cardiovascular diseases.

Such studies can be deceptive, however. Women who choose to take hormones after menopause may be healthier, or have other health behaviors that would reduce their risk of heart disease, even if they weren't taking hormones. In order to really determine whether hormones protect the heart, a different kind of study needed to be done.

These other studies, called "clinical trials," compared two groups of women who are the same in all characteristics. One group received hormone treatment and the other, a placebo (dummy pill). These new studies *did not* show hormone treat-ment to be beneficial in protecting women from heart disease. In fact, not only was there *no* benefit; there was also a slight, but important, increase in the risk for heart attack, stroke, blood clots in the lungs and breast cancer. What it adds up to is that at this time there is no evidence to support the use of hormones after menopause to prevent heart disease.

Today, hormones are indicated *only* as treatment for the uncomfortable symptoms of menopause, and they should be used for the shortest possible time. The best way to prevent heart disease during and after menopause is by identifying and treating risk factors such as high blood pressure, high cholesterol, smoking, diabetes, lack of exercise and obesity.

At this time there is no evidence to support the use of hormones after menopause to prevent heart disease.

Menopause is an important life change. Some women take it in stride and flourish, while others are distressed by it. But however a woman may react to it, menopause is an inescapable fact of life and women live 25–30% of their lives after menopause. So learn all you can about it, talk to your doctor, and learn how best to manage your health during this period. It's in your power to make menopause a positive experience, by learning how to stay healthy now and for a long time after.

CHAPTER 13

HOW SPIRITUALITY CAN HELP YOUR CARDIOVASCULAR HEALTH

The spirituality of African American women is associated with a variety of positive health outcomes. The traditional definition of spirituality involves one's acknowledgement of, and relationship to, a Supreme Being, supernatural force or creator of all things. Religion, related to spirituality, refers to religious attendance, practice or activity.

As African American women, we're likely to involve ourselves in spiritual/religious activities, such as church attendance, prayer, healing, meditation, devotion, affirmation, religious experience, and ritual. These are resources we use to meet the daily spiritual needs of our families and ourselves. Spirituality and religion have always played a strong part in the health of African American women.

Religious practice and the sense of community it brings help protect us from stresses that might otherwise get us down and even make us ill. It's also true that, within the African American community, houses of worship not only provide emotional support but they can and do become centers for health awareness.

If your church isn't already a health aware community, or, if it *is* but wants to become even more involved, see Dr. Kristen L. Mauk's *Congregational Health: How to Make Your Congregation a Health-Aware Community* (Hilton Publishing: Roscoe, IL, 2003) and *A Minute for Your Health*, edited for The Association of Black Cardiologists by Stephanie H. Kong, M.D. (Hilton Publishing: Roscoe, IL., 2003). Both are useful handbooks for getting started.

The idea that the spiritual self and physical self are tightly connected has found validation and interest in health sciences. For instance, The World Health Organization (WHO) defines health as one's physical, emotional, and spiritual/religious state of being. Studies show that spirituality can influence self-esteem and a sense of belonging, and that it can also encourage the right kind of attention to our bodies and our health. Some tests find that spirituality is associated with lower blood pressure, better immune function, and decreased depression.

Spirituality contributes to better health by providing us with important coping skills. It helps us to love and to interpret our social relationships compassionately. It gives order and meaning to our daily lives. It graces us with peace, comfort, and hope. Those qualities together are a firm foundation for good health habits. When we feel right about ourselves and about others, we're most likely to work at staying healthy.

For many African American women, the quality that holds all the others together is faith. Our faith is defined within a cultural context and directly relates to our cultural belief system. Within this system, our faith strengthens family and community relationships, and it teaches us, collectively and as individuals, to experience power in all our daily activities.

Two Medicines

Historically, spirituality for African Americans stems from African spiritual traditions. These traditions acknowledge all living things and honor ancestors as current influences on our lives. During slavery, there was a deliberate attempt to destroy African culture. But despite the oppression, African Americans transcended and transformed these experiences through spirituality.

Spirituality gave our ancestors hope and coping mechanisms to combat the terrible pressures within the family and community relationships that slavery imposed. During this time, gospel music was born, and circuit preachers made their rounds. Further, African Americans learned to hold forums aimed at organizing for mutual benefit, coming up with strategies for freedom, and bringing about change and improvement of their place in American life.

African American women played a central part during this era and after. They were the healers, nurturers and educators of the generations to come. They brought about the movement from African religions to Christian ones. But at least one aspect of the old religion survived the change. For African Americans, interpretations of illness and disease often included the spiritual dimension.

Until quite recently, spirituality and healing were inseparable. In some cultures, the priest and physician was the same person, administering spiritual and physical health with divine sanction. But the popularity of scientific (Western) medicine in the middle 19th century separated medicine from spirituality and religion completely. The priest and physician were no longer one and the same.

In spite of that division, things seem to be changing again. Some of that change depends on scientific research. For example, R.C. Byrd in 1988 reported over 35 studies indicating that prayers and meditations could be beneficial for individuals at a distance by relieving stress. (As we know, high levels of stress contribute to increased risk for developing many illnesses including cardiovascular disease.) More recent studies seem to support this claim that group prayer can give a better chance to cardiac-care unit patients. Although we need more studies in this area, we can at least say that evidence is showing that prayer and other forms of spiritual intervention can help our healing.

Of course, this works in the other direction too. Churches and other faith-based institutions are especially well positioned to encourage better health in our community, because they are grounded in social support and community outreach. The message they can pass along is that, in ways that are still mysterious to us, the life of the spirit and the life of the body are one life. Communities that realize this will work to bring preventive medicine and basic medical information to their congregations. They know that the improvement of individual and community health can increase our quality of life. They also know that, should we fall ill, our life in the spirit can improve our chances of getting well. Further, although religion and spirituality may not prevent illness directly, they help us to cope more effectively with life's pressures. One survey reports that 90% of the general population says they pray and 80% believe that prayer heals.

In any case, science is just beginning to tell us what we have known all along. When we enter the spiritual realm, we understand that we don't control all aspects of our lives. Giving up that control where appropriate gives us some relief that we do not carry burdens alone. The spirit lightens our burdens.

That is the message that we African American women are well suited to pass on to our children. We all know that women are the glue of the community and that they shape the reality our children experience and the way they see the world. Let's not miss the chance to teach our children the spiritual and medical truths that can give them healthy and happy lives.

In summary, what you should now know about heart disease is: twice as many women have heart disease than have cancer, and the number of deaths that result from heart disease is more than double the number caused by all forms of cancer together. Bringing it home, African American women and other women of color are more likely to die from their heart disease than other women. Heart disease is preventable if you know your risk factors and work with your healthcare professional to reduce these risks. The risk of heart disease in African American children can be reduced by mothers taking charge of family health, providing healthy meals and encouraging an active lifestyle.

The task is our own, individual by individual. We hope the whole community will begin to understand the basic medical facts this book offers. We hope everyone will see a doctor or provider regularly. And we also hope that people spread the word about the power of spirituality to strengthen your health. Only then can we hope to reverse an epidemic of poor heart health that threatens our community.

Learn and teach, keep yourself and your children and your loved ones on the path to heart healthiness.

PART III

Negotiating the
Health Care System

CHAPTER 14

WORKING WITH PROVIDERS

Medicine in the 21st century is going through a time of exciting discoveries about the causes and treatment of diseases. Life expectancy has increased dramatically over the twentieth century. Further, technology exists today that lets physicians diagnose many diseases very precisely and at earlier stages of the disease, both of which increase the likelihood of a cure or successful disease management. We know more about disease prevention than ever in the history of mankind. All this makes medicine an exciting and ever-changing field that brings new benefits to patients.

But some bare truths about medicine aren't likely to change, regardless of the technology. For example, unless a woman takes her own health and her family's health into her hands, all the diagnostic tools, preventative strategies and medicines won't help her, because she won't know how to get to them. Far too many African American women are in exactly that situation now.

Instead of regularly seeing doctors and other healthcare providers, we too often depend on emergency rooms at the local hospital. That way of getting healthcare is dangerous. First, many people seek care in this setting when disease symptoms have become severe, and diseases are at advanced stages. Too many people don't get medical attention until it is too late. The second problem with emergency rooms is that they aren't set up to do follow up or preventative care. Health needs to be monitored regularly so that women, working with healthcare providers, can take whatever health steps are needed in order to prevent disease and increase wellness.

Your choice of doctor is also very important. Not all primary care doctors are created equal. In your search for a primary care doctor, don't be taken in by gender, race, creed or a beautifully decorated office. Even information about how well educated a certain doctor may be doesn't necessarily mean that this is the right doctor for you.

Beyond having a solid medical education, with three or more years training beyond medical school, a good doctor has a real thirst for the detective work necessary for proper diagnosis, and keeps up with the newest discoveries in medicine. A good doctor will also counsel you and monitor disease prevention strategies to ensure the best quality of life. Finally, a good doctor has genuine respect for his or her patients and wants to help them.

You'll want a doctor who takes time with you. His or her patience makes him or her better able to diagnose a complex disease process and to take the very best care of you.

While these are the qualities you want in a doctor, you don't always get them. Too often "members" of an Health Maintenance Organization (HMO) and private patients are short-changed just when they most need a careful examination. HMOs seem more and more driven solely by profit, so doctors are driven harder and harder to see a high number of patients each day. That means the doctor has less time to work with you and gives you less attention.

In recent years, there have been lawsuits against doctors and HMOs that caused damage through hasty exams. A better course is for you, as an African American woman, to understand the careful and thorough exam you need, and to insist on it. Your knowledge also helps ensure that you select the right provider.

How Do You Select a Doctor?

How you select your doctor is as important as how you select your mate. If you belong to an HMO, you may not get a wide list of doctors. So talk with people in the same HMO, people you trust, and ask whether they're satisfied with their providers, and why. Good common sense tells people whether or not they are in the care of someone who genuinely cares about them and their health.

When you go in for a first meeting with a health-care provider, take family members or reliable friends with you. Their opinions may help you make your choice. Even if your HMO doesn't allow you to decide which doctor you get, the more you already understand about your health, the more you will be empowered to insist on proper health monitoring.

Although some HMOs don't allow you to choose your doctor, most allow you to choose your kind of doctor. In making that choice, here is what you need to know.

All states have a Board of Medical Examiner's office that gathers statistics and keeps records of disciplinary actions against doctors licensed to practice in that state. Many states have internet access to the data they collect. This is a reasonable place to start to check out a doctor you are considering or one to whom you've been assigned. If there is a pattern of, or multiple cases of, malpractice suits against the doctor you are considering, you should insist on a different provider.

Doctors have different levels of training. You may wish to ask your medical provider which of the following categories she fits into.

Board Certification refers to the testing that a physician has undergone to prove competency. In order to be Board Certified, a physician must undergo several years of training after medical school and pass a difficult test of knowledge.

Board Eligible means that the physician has all of the training required in that specialty or subspecialty but has either not taken the board exam for that specialty or has not passed the exam.

WHAT TYPE OF DOCTOR TO SELECT

The answer depends on the state of your current health and whether your health-care needs are simple or complicated. All adults need a primary care provider. If you are over forty, or if you are younger but have a complex medical history, you may be best served by having a general internist or adult medicine specialist. If you are young and healthy and want the same doctor for your children as well as yourself, a family practitioner may serve your needs best.

Internal Medicine Specialists (or *Internists*) are trained for three years, sometimes four, at certified residency programs in the care of adults seventeen years and older. In training adult medicine specialists, intense attention is paid to each of the internal organ systems of the body. Internists are also trained in the care and treatment of very sick people.

Training as an internist is necessary for any doctor who wants to practice specialized medicine, such as cardiology (heart specialist), rheumatology (joint specialist), pulmonary (lung specialist), and many others.

Family Practice is an emerging field for care across the entire lifespan. Ideally, becoming a family practitioner requires three years of training at a certified residency program that focuses on the care of pregnant women, infants, children, adolescents, and adults. However, as a rule in these programs, the amount of specific training in organ systems is reduced and so is intensive care training

The family practitioner can be especially helpful in rural settings where there are few doctors, and for young people and mature people in good health, who don't need complicated treatment and care. People of any age who have complex symptoms, or a history of life-threatening illness, or multiple medical conditions may be better served by general internists for their primary care.

Many women, especially those younger than fifty, may use an obstetrician/gynecologist as their primary care giver. These are physicians trained in all aspects of women's reproductive health. Because so many young women see only OB/Gyn physicians, many of these physicians also do all of the routine health maintenance for their young women patients.

Doctors in *General Practice* are a dying breed. GPs (General Practitioners) have gone through medical school but they have had only one additional year of limited training. "GPs" are usu-ally not considered well enough trained to serve as primary care providers in HMOs and other systems of organized medicine.

Primary care providers (whether internists, family practition-ers, obstetricians/gynecologists, or pediatricians) serve as gate-keepers for specialists in most managed care organizations. What that means is that they decide whether to allow you to seek spe-cialized care and how long you can keep going to the specialists once you've begun. You will need a primary care provider (PCP) even if you are under treatment for a specific disease, such as dia-betes or thyroid dysfunction. The primary care provider ensures not only that you get necessary treatment, but also that you learn and practice the best ways to stay well.

Why Go to Your doctor When You Feel Healthy?

The answer is simple: for the same reason you get a tune-up on your car or check the oil after so many miles. Learning and prac-ticing good health habits and early detection are the keys to pre-venting or surviving many poten-tially devastating illnesses before they can do damage! A once-yearly physical exam is highly rec-ommended for adults starting at age forty even if you are in excel-lent health.

Learning and practicing good health habits and early detection are the keys to preventing or surviving many potentially devastating illnesses before they can do damage!

The yearly exam is a good time for women to have a mammogram and Pap smear, and for men to have a prostate exam and to determine cardiovascular risk. Such exams save lives. The yearly visit can help your doctor update your own medical history and your family's. It also gives your doctor the opportunity to examine your organ systems, with the help of lab work.

For women who want to stay healthy, there's nothing more important than the yearly physical exam. Even if you don't have insurance, you can probably work out with your doctor fees and scheduled payments that suit your income.

YOUR MEDICAL HISTORY

At an annual visit or first visit with a new health-care provider, your provider will first want to hear about your own, and your family's, health history, going back to parents and even grandparents. Your doctor should ask about any complaints you may have, your allergies, medications, habits, social history, family history, and past medical and surgical history. If the doctor doesn't ask the question, simply remind him or her by reading them from a list you've written down and brought with you.

Some serious diseases run in families. So your doctor needs to get from you the best information on your parents' health, even if they are now deceased. Keep in mind that the purpose of such questions is to *ensure your good health*. Sometimes, on the basis of family history, your provider can steer you to a prevention program that keeps you from developing a certain disease.

Your doctor will want to know what medicines you're taking, so bring in the list you've prepared with the names of the medicines and the dosage. (If you are using non-prescription drugs or herbal/natural remedies, put these on the list as well.) Keep that list in a safe place in your purse, like a wallet. That way, if you're in an accident and can't speak, the list will give to people who treat you information they need. Some of us simply don't like to deal with lists, and that's OK. Just bring the medicine bottles with you in your shopping bag.

Your doctor needs to know about any previous medical problems or surgery you may have had, including the year of the diagnosis or operation. Before your appointment, write this history down. Sometimes it's easier to remember such things when we're comfortable at home than it is in the doctor's office. It's helpful if you have notes to work from when the doctor asks the questions. Besides, by writing down your health history, you will gain a better understanding of the state of your own health and will be well on your way to entering a partnership with your doctor, whose mission is your best health. You may be surprised to find out how good it feels to take on the responsibility of your own and your family's health.

Naturally, a good partnership means working with a doctor you respect and trust. If your doctor doesn't listen to you, or doesn't take time to explain himself to you in clear language that you understand, look for another one.

A reliable physical exam depends on your being unrobed. Never accept an examination through your clothes. Do not be shy about having your clothes off. Just remember why it is necessary. Both heart and breath sounds are muffled through your clothes, so they don't give your doctor the information he needs. It's also true that abdominal tumors or other abnormalities are harder to find through clothing. Even socks can be a problem. People with diabetes sometimes get ulcers on the toe or foot that could lead to amputation of a limb, yet these people may not feel pain in the affected areas, because of the way the disease has

---

The Physical Exam

A complete physical exam can only properly be done while you are disrobed. The physical exam looks at the following parts and systems of your body:

- Eyes
- Ears
- Mouth
- Neck
- Chest
- Breast
- Heart

- Abdomen
- Genitalia
- Rectum
- Extremities
- Neurologic system
- Musculoskeletal system

---

injured nerves to the feet and legs. Your doctor can find these ulcers usually at an early stage, when successful treatment is still possible.

When you go in for your physical exam, it's a good idea to take along a spouse, significant other, or friend (particularly one who knows something about health care). This is especially true if you believe you may have a serious disease. During the visit, you may feel anxious and even afraid. Your friend or spouse will be in a better position to take notes during your talk with your doctor, after the physical exam is complete. Later, the notes will tell you

- What the doctor said about diagnosis
- Whether you will need further tests

- What treatment plan, if you need one, the doctor recommended
- The date of your next visit

GETTING YOUR DOCTOR'S ATTENTION

Too many providers dismiss women's health complaints as unimportant and tend to give men more attention. That's why you need to be as clear as you can about what you are feeling and why it worries you. It is your right to have a doctor who listens. The elderly, too, must know their medical rights, since doctors also tend to give them less attention.

Many of us meet open bias on a daily basis. These biases sometimes influence a doctor's thinking about diagnosis and treatment. For example, that bias is likely to show when an emotionally distressed African American woman presents herself for diagnosis and possible treatment. Be sure your doctor explains to you, in language you can clearly understand, why he or she thinks you have an emotional disease.

Sometimes you can help yourself when you're not getting the right respect from your health-care provider or you suspect that you're not getting a good examination or the right treatment. Just mention your cousin, the lawyer. Often, that's enough to get your doctor's attention and keep it.

Here's an amusing anecdote. It began when a modest-appearing African American family came to a world famous medical institution to try to get care for their daughter, who had Type 1 (childhood onset) diabetes.

As a doctor in training at this institution, I noticed that every doctor who worked with them had special respect for this family, and worked hard to provide the best possible care for the daughter. I noticed also that in discussing the case these doctors would inevitably remark: "You know, her brother is an attorney!"

One day when I happened to be "on call," I had a chance to talk with the family. They let me know that they'd invented the attorney! They'd noticed before that her daughter got better care if they mentioned this fictional relative. Mr. Willie Gary and Johnny Cochrane have lots of relatives!

If you or a friend has relatives who *are* doctors or healthcare professionals, you might ask them to call your doctor for a discussion of your serious, or potentially serious, health issues.

GETTING WHAT YOU DESERVE FROM HMOs

You may not be able to change the system, but you *can* do a few things that ensure the right kind of care for you and your family. The HMO system is no place for shrinking violets. If you are not getting what you believe you need, you must complain to the powers that be, up to and including, the medical director.

Even during your physical, be on your toes, and politely insist that you get *all* the features of a physical exam. Doctors may not wish to prescribe specialized treatments, such as, for example, colonoscopy. They may, in fact, be encouraged not to recommend certain treatments, by payments and rewards from the HMOs for saving money at *your* health's expense!

> *If you are not getting what you believe you need, you must complain to the powers that be, up to and including, the medical director.*

HMOs don't block all specialized treatments. For example, because breast cancer is so emotionally charged and, as a woman's health issue, is highly politicized, pretty much all HMO institutions provide good treatment for this cancer, and allow patients medical visits to determine the success of the treatment and to give them the support they need.

Colon cancer, on the other hand, isn't always treated so generously, even though colon cancer is more widespread than breast cancer, and more deadly. Colon cancer has few reliable early warning symptoms. This means that the patient who has it may not know she is ill until it's too late.

With proper medical attention, colon cancer is more preventable than breast cancer. But HMOs are reluctant to provide the proper screening and treatment. The standard of care for colon cancer screening is colonoscopy. But too often HMOs don't cover this procedure because it is more costly than less reliable procedures. That's why you must insist on colonoscopy if you are fifty years old or more, and earlier if you have a family history of colon cancer or if you have other diseases of the colon. Take that responsibility. It can save your life. As we say, patients need to take the initiative. Your life is too important to be run by fear.

Your particular physical exam will be specific to you, the fact that you are a woman, your age, and lifestyle. Problems a doctor looks for in a twenty-three year-old woman are very different from the ones he'd look for in a woman of seventy. But all physical exams have common elements, as described above.

WHAT YOU NEED TO KNOW ABOUT TAKING MEDICINES

Your doctor may prescribe medication. Talk to the doctor about how the generic (or common) version of the medication stands up against the brand name. Generic drugs are cheaper, and they often are as effective as trade-name drugs. But in some specific cases, generic drugs *don't* work as well. A good doctor will know when and which to prescribe.

Once you've started taking medication, be sure to monitor it. For instance, if your blood pressure rises or diabetic control worsens, your pharmacy may have substituted a generic drug for the brand-name prescribed by your doctor. Discuss this with your pharmacist and physician. It is essential that you fill your prescription and take the medication as prescribed.

Self-Medicating

Self-medicating is very dangerous, although many people do it. Of course, occasionally using a pill to reduce fever or as an antacid usually causes no problem. But if you are using a non-prescription medicine regularly, be sure to tell your doctor. At the same time, don't start taking a prescription drug regularly without talking to your doctor.

Self-medicating with narcotic pain pills is especially dangerous. If your pain is so great that you feel you need to take a narcotic pain pill that has not been prescribed for this condition, you need to see your physician immediately. Pain is a very efficient warning system that something is wrong with your body. If you interfere with that warning system by medicating with narcotics, you can create a problem with devastating consequences!

EMERGENCY ROOM CARE

Sometimes there are long waits in emergency rooms. People with chest pains and people brought in by ambulance generally get seen most quickly. If you do have to wait, be patient. You've gotten to the place where you can get the best possible diagnosis and treatment for your potentially serious medical condition. This means lab work, EKG, and chest x-rays, with follow up. While the ER may be the appropriate place for care when new symptoms suddenly appear, the downside of emergency room care is that you do not establish a relationship with a particular physician who gets to know all of your health related facts. Very often, emergency room care is focused on the single problem you complained of, with little attention paid to other health issues. Preventative care is *never* addressed in the ER.

WORKING WITH YOUR PROVIDER IF YOU'RE HOSPITALIZED

If you are hospitalized in a teaching hospital (that is, a hospital affiliated with a medical school), you may be cared for by students from the earliest to the most advanced stages of their education. Insist that you and your family speak with the attending M.D. (the supervising doctor who is in charge of your case) and R.N. (registered nurse) so they are aware there is family support. That way, the doctor and nurse will know they are accountable.

If you're hospitalized, you may run into a kind of doctor known as *Hospitalists*. The notion here is that doctors who take care of hospitalized patients exclusively can do so with more efficiency and at less cost than the office-based primary care doctor. The patient's problem is that, for Hospitalists, early discharge is the rule rather than the exception. If you don't feel ready to be discharged when the hospital says you should, get a relative to call your provider and to insist on knowing the reason for the early discharge. If you are discharged early, before you can take care of yourself, *insist* on home care, unless you have responsible relatives willing and able to provide it.

LONG-TERM NURSING CARE

Long-term care, or "nursing home" care, has flourished in this country for several decades (such institutions were once called "rest homes"). In the past, nursing homes provided care only for the elderly, but today they also serve young and severely incapacitated patients. Because patients in such care are predominately elderly people close to the end of their lives, they don't always get the care they deserve. Too many nursing homes look after their patients simply by feeding them and responding to their most basic needs.

Bedsores can cause great discomfort for older patients. Worse still, bedsores can create the environment for an infection that even gets into the bloodstream and is hard to cure. Nursing staffs can prevent bedsores by turning patients regularly, so that no one part of the body gets severely irritated. *The presence or absence of bedsores is a barometer of the quality of care the nursing home provides.*

If you or a family member resides in a nursing home, keep a close eye on whether caregivers are responsive to the patient's needs and that they move bed-ridden patients often enough to prevent falls and bedsores.

HOSPICE CARE[1]

Patients who have only six months or less to live will often be provided with hospice care, at home or in a hospital or nursing home. Hospice assistance can give great comfort. The service also provides strong spiritual support to the patient and to the family after the death occurs. The hospice's volunteer staff is made up of registered nurses (RNs) and other trained volunteers. Everyone on the hospice staff is skilled at pain management, symptom control, and bereavement assistance. A team assigned to a particular patient usually includes a doctor, but often the doctor plays little direct part in the care.

Hospice is a federally funded Medicare benefit offered to a dying person, the person's family, and loved ones. Hospice staff makes the dying patient more comfortable, with up-to-date supportive and pain relief measures. They also can help families manage home care, and help ease them through this difficult time.

Most terminally ill people (85% according to a recent Gallup poll) would prefer to die in their homes with loved ones around them. Hospice can help make that a reality.

To be eligible for Hospice services a patient must be declared to have six months or less to live. Terminal cancer patients are often referred to hospice care, as are very debilitated, elderly patients such as stroke victims.

Here is a complete list of services offered by the Medicare Hospice Benefit Organization:

---

1. The material in this section draws on *Taking Care of Our Own*, by G. Edmond Smith, MD, M.Ed. (Hilton Publishing, 2003)

- Visits by the multidisciplinary team to hospitals (hospice may sometimes have their own wards or hospital floors), homes, and nursing homes
- Rental or purchase of durable medical equipment
- Payment for supplies ordered by the hospice team
- Payment for drugs used in palliative care (in some instances, the family pays a minimal co-payment)
- Shared management with the doctor of all aspects of care for the terminally ill patient
- Necessary social services by staff social workers
- Counseling for dietary needs, bereavement, and pastoral care
- Physical, occupational, and speech therapy

One warning: hospices will commonly use morphine to ease the pain of their patients. If you decide to use hospice for yourself or a loved one, talk over the morphine question. Morphine use can hasten death.

REHABILITATION HOSPITAL CARE

Rehabilitation centers provide physical therapy or speech therapy to patients who have had strokes or surgery and who are unable to walk and get around. Typically, insurance companies allow only a few weeks of such therapy. Often they are discharged before they are ready to go home. But these centers will recommend follow-up exercises and practice that that the patient can do at home.

SUMMING UP

Taking charge of your health requires two big choices:

1. the choice to embrace a healthy lifestyle
2. the choice to become an active and informed partner with your physician in screening, diagnosing and treating illness.

What you've read in this book is what you need to know to work with the health system. Here's to your good health!

A HEALTH CHECK-UP LIST FOR AFRICAN AMERICAN WOMEN

- TEETH: See your dentist every six months for a standard cleaning.

- DIABETES: If you are at risk, consult your physician. You should expect a sugar test at the time of the yearly physical.

- SMOKING: Discuss how to quit smoking. Talk to your doctor about options.

- BLOOD: Blood count and cholesterol should be tested at your routine physical.

- CHOLESTEROL TEST: Begin at age 18 and continue every five years, unless your provider recommends a more frequent schedule.

- BLOOD PRESSURE READING: All children should be tested for blood pressure during yearly health visits. Start getting readings at 18, and continue to do so every one or two years. If blood pressure is abnormal, a plan to reduce it should be initiated and blood pressure checks should be more frequent.

- IMMUNIZATIONS: Tetanus-Diphtheria Booster, Flu Shot, and Tuberculin Test. If over 60 or have chronic lung disease or disease decreasing immune function, a pneumonia vaccine.

- SKIN: Consult your doctor if you have any unusual brown spots, bumps, sores, rashes, or moles.

- ABDOMEN: Make sure that your your doctor checks for enlargement of the spleen or liver at your yearly physicals.

- FEET: If you're at risk for diabetes, consult your physician to advise you on foot care.

- KNEES: A knee reflex test screens for neuromuscular disease.

- UNDERARMS: Your doctor will check for lymph nodes.

- BREAST SELF-EXAM: Begin at age 20 and continue once a month.

- BREAST EXAM BY A TRAINED HEALTHCARE PROFESSIONAL: Begin at age 25 and continue every three years until age 39; continue annually if you are age 40 or older.

- MAMMOGRAM: Begin at age 35 and continue every one to two years until age 50. After 50, you should have a mammogram every year.

- Pelvic Exam, including a Pap Smear Test: Begin at age 18 or at the onset of sexual activity, if earlier, and continue annually.

- Sexually transmitted disease (STD) screening: Begin when you become sexually active.

- Colon cancer screening: Begin at age 50 and continue once a year. If you have a family history of colon cancer or polyps (small growths in the colon that are a risk factor for colon cancer) or other intestinal diseases, you should begin having regular screenings at a younger age. Ask your health care professional for guidance.

- Bone Mineral Density Exam & Bone mass measurement: This screening is typically first given in a woman's 40s, and then repeated annually after menopause.

QUESTIONS TO
ASK YOUR DOCTOR

One key to working well with your doctor is asking the right questions. Here are examples of questions to ask your doctor during your annual physical, or by phone if you have concerns:

HEART DISEASE AND STROKE

1. What are the symptoms of heart disease and stroke?
2. What tests should I have, and how often, to monitor my risk factors for developing heart disease and stroke?
3. What do my test results mean? Do I have heart disease?
4. What sort of treatment plan do you recommend?
5. Can you help me plan a safe exercise program?
6. Am I at high risk for heart-related complications if I take birth control pills?
7. What are the possible side effects of medications I've been prescribed?

8. What should I do if I experience chest pains or other symptoms of angina or heart attack?
9. How can I distinguish angina from a heart attack?
10. I'm confused about hormone replacement therapy (HRT). Can you help me understand the most recent discussions about HRT and heart disease?
11. How can I change my diet—including the addition of vitamins—to improve my cardiovascular health?
12. Should I take aspirin as a preventative therapy? If so, how much and how often?

HIGH BLOOD PRESSURE

1. What is my current risk for developing hypertension? What is my future risk?
2. Am I taking any medicines that make me more susceptible to hypertension?
3. How can I limit my risk and help prevent hypertension?
4. What medications are available to help me if I have hypertension? What are their benefits and side effects?
5. Will these drugs interact with any other medications I am taking?
6. What are the symptoms of hypertension?
7. What does my blood pressure reading mean?
8. How will we know which medication is best for me?
9. My blood pressure is only slightly above normal. Do I really have to do anything about it?
10. Is there a cure for hypertension?
11. For the person with high blood pressure: Is there evi-

dence of damage to any organ or system–kidneys, heart, or brain?

12. If I have high blood pressure are my children at risk also?

CHOLESTEROL

1. When should I schedule a cholesterol test?
2. What do the test results mean?
3. What steps should I take to lower my cholesterol?
4. When should I have a follow-up test?
5. How does food influence cholesterol?
6. My cholesterol is high. Should I be taking a cholesterol-reducing drug?
7. If I have high blood cholesterol are my children at risk also?
8. What are the side effects of the medications I'm taking? Does it make any difference what time of day I take them?
9. Can you recommend a good registered dietitian with a track record in helping women reduce their cholesterol levels?
10. I have diabetes. How does that change our approach to treating high cholesterol.

SMOKING

1. How is my (or my partner's) smoking affecting my health?
2. How can I quit smoking? Should I use a nicotine replacement therapy or other medicines?

3. What will be the health effects if I don't stop smoking?

4. Is my (or my partner's) smoking affecting my children's health?

5. What are the health benefits of quitting smoking now?

6. Do you have any "stop smoking" literature available for me to take home and read?

7. Why have I been unsuccessful in my attempts to quit smoking in the past? What can I learn from those experiences?

8. Should my partner and I quit smoking together? What if he or she won't quit with me?

9. What are the effects of second-hand smoke? How can I limit my exposure to second-hand smoke?

10. What kinds of withdrawal symptoms should I expect? How can I cope with them?

OBESITY

1. Have my body composition and risk factors—as well as my height and weight—been considered in your diagnosis?

2. Based on my current weight and eating patterns and goal weight, how many calories a day should I eat in my weight loss efforts?

3. How will I be evaluated to determine if I am an appropriate candidate for appetite suppressant medication treatment?

4. What other medical conditions or medications might

influence my decision to take an appetite suppressant medication?

5. What type of program will be provided along with the medication to help me improve my eating and physical activity habits?

6. Am I a candidate for obesity surgery? Why or why not?

7. What are the complications or possible side effects of any type of diet, medication, surgery, or other treatment you are recommending? What symptoms should I watch for?

8. How can I maintain weight loss?

FITNESS

1. What are the best types of exercises for me? How should I tailor my exercise program to my particular fitness needs?

2. Based on my fitness level, how much and what types of exercise would be best for me to start with?

3. Do I need to undergo an electrocardiography or other type of test before beginning an exercise program? What is my resting heart rate? What should my heart rate be while I'm exercising?

4. What symptoms should I be concerned with while I'm exercising?

5. At what duration, frequency and intensity should I begin my exercise program? What should I be able to work up to?

6. What if I experience chest pain, faintness or dizziness, bone or joint pain while exercising?

7. If weight training is recommended, what weight should I start out with?

8. How might my medications affect my exercise program, especially exercise intensity and heart rate response?

9. Should I change my diet in any way after I start an exercise program?

10. Can you recommend a hospital-based fitness program?

WEIGHT MANAGEMENT

1. How will I be evaluated to determine if I am underweight, at a normal weight or overweight?

2. Will my fitness level or body composition be taken into consideration when you make that determination?

3. Could any medical conditions I have or medications I am taking affect my weight management efforts, and in what ways?

4. What risk factors do I have for diseases due to being overweight? How do my risk factors come into play?

5. What type of complications or side effects have been reported for any sort of special diet plan or supplement you are recommending?

6. What are the best types of exercises for me? How should I tailor my exercise program to my particular fitness needs?

7. Can you recommend a hospital-based weight-management program or a nutritionist or registered dietitian who can help me put together a healthy eating plan?

Stress

1. Could I have an underlying medical condition that could be causing my symptoms?
2. Could some medication I'm taking be causing my symptoms?
3. Has my stress caused physical or mental illness that needs to be dealt with medically, separately from the stress itself?
4. If the stress is left untreated, what will happen to my health?
5. Can you refer me to a mental health professional who can teach me how to best manage and control my stress?
6. Can you teach me various relaxation techniques or refer me to someone who can?
7. Can you refer me to an effective stress management workshop?
8. What other techniques or resources can you tell me about?

Diabetes

1. Is my blood sugar normal?
2. How often should it be tested?
3. If you have diabetes, is my A, C test at target?
4. Can you refer me to a nutritionist to plan and understand my diet?
5. What tests do I need to monitor for diabetic damage to my eyes, heart, nerves and circulation?
6. What kind and how much exercise is safe for me?

7. What medications do I need? Explain what they do and what their side effects are.
8. If I have diabetes are my children at risk also?
9. Help me understand how to manage my diabetes when I'm pregnant.

APPENDIX C

RESOURCES TO HELP YOU

T he *Association of Black Cardiologists Center for Women's Health* offers a video "Heart Health for the Generations," the Generations program for women, and other instructional material on heart disease prevention, treatment and research specifically directed to the African American community. www.abcardio.org

American Heart Association: funds heart disease medical research tudies and offers comprehensive information about various heart conditions and treatments. Sponsors an excellent public education campaign for women about heart disease, *"Taking Wellness to Heart."* Call toll-free 888–MY–HEART for the campaign's FREE educational materials.

Agency for Healthcare Research and Quality: (AHRQ) publishes a series of comprehensive Clinical Practice Guidelines on heart disease (and other medical conditions) by panels of leading medical experts. These reports describe the best current knowledge and treatment guidelines for doctors and health care professionals to follow. (They are good reference guides especially if you think you may not be getting the best medical care available.) Less technical Patient and Family Guides are also available for each of the following reports:

- Heart Failure: Patients with Left-Ventricular Systolic Dysfunction
- Unstable Angina: Diagnosis and Management
- Cardiac Rehabilitation

You may download these documents from the AHRQ's Web site at www.ahcpr.gov/ or order them for free by calling toll free 800–358–9295.

Black Women's Health Imperative (BWHI): Black Women's Health Imperative, the new name of the National Black Women's Health Project, is a leading African American health education, research, advocacy and leadership development institution.

Walking for Wellness Program: The National Black Women's Health Imperatives exercise program. promotes healthy lifestyles and disease prevention through encouraging Black women to walk and talk in groups. Contact: www.blackwomenshealth.org

Smoking Cessation Programs: Stop smoking programs are offered in your community by the American Lung Association (call

800–242–8721) and the American Cancer Society (call 800–227–2345).

HeartCenterOnline: an on-line resource for information and news about heart disease, risk factors, treatments, and patients' stories. You can also sign up for their free weekly E-mail newsletter devoted to heart disease and treatments. Contact: www.heartcenteronline.com

Heart Information Network: offers comprehensive information on heart disease. Especially helpful are its *Q&A Library* and *Glossary*, which explains medical jargon. http://www.heart info.org/

Heartmates: an organization offering online support to spouses and family members of people with heart disease. It's geared more for wives of men with heart disease but still offers good advice, videos on recovery, and a helpful book, *Heartmates: A Guide for the Spouse and Family of the Heart Patient. Contact: www.heartmates.com/* Phone 612–558–3331.

Mended Hearts: affiliated with the American Heart Association, this national network of support groups is for people recovering from heart bypass surgery and other procedures. Call 1–888–HEART99 (1–888–432–7899) to see about talking to a heart patient in your area.

National Heart, Lung and Blood Institute (NHBLI) of the National Institutes of Health: funds medical research and provides expert information on all aspects of heart disease, including women and heart disease. Call 301–592–8573 to order its free packet of fact sheets on women and heart disease. Also, call toll free 800–575–9355 to hear recorded information (in English and Spanish) about high blood pressure and high cholesterol treatments. NHLBI also sponsors a *National Heart Attack Alert Program and the Heart Truth Campaign focused on heart disease in women.* http://www.nhlbi.nih.gov/health/hearttruth/index.htm.

WomenHeart: The National Coalition for Women with Heart Disease: WomenHeart was founded by three women who had heart attacks while in their 40s and faced many obstacles, including misdiagnosis and social isolation. They were each amazed how little information about or services for women with heart disease were available, and also how the issue seemed invisible within the women's health community. Contact: www.womenheart.org/

ADDITIONAL RESOURCES

Many insurance companies have health promotion and disease prevention programs. These companies will offer health education classes free of charge. Check with your health insurance provider for a list of classes.

Here is a guide of still other available resources:

Church Programs: Check your and other churches in your community for health promoting programs.

YWCA and YMCA programs: Call your local YWCA or YMCA. Many offer health programs and may also offer child care.

American Diabetes Association (ADA)
Alexandria, VA; 1–703–549–1500
1–800–DIABETES
ADA offers free publications and sells books on diabetes.
www.diabetes.org

American Dietetic Association
1–800–366–1655
Provides nutrition information and referrals to local registered
dietitians
www.eatright.org

American Heart Association
Dallas, Texas 1–800–242–8721
Offers free brochures such as "About High Blood Pressure in
African Americans."
www.americanheart.org

American Kidney Fund
Rockville, Md; 1–800–638–8299
Ask for the free brochure, "African Americans and High Blood
Pressure."
www.kidneyfund.org

American Medical Women's Association
Alexandria, Va; 1–703–838–0500
Offers "Guide to Healthy Eating" and other free information
www.amwa-doc.org

American Stroke Association
1–888–4STROKE (1–888–478–7653)
A division of the American Heart Association
www.StrokeAssociation.org

Association of Black Cardiologists (ABC)
Atlanta, GA; 1–678–302–4222
ABC was founded in 1974 to bring special attention to the adverse impact of cardiovascular disease on African Americans
www.abcardio.org

Association of Black Psychologists
Washington, DC 1–202–722–0808
www.abpsi.org

Calorie Control Council
Atlanta, GA
Offers free information on weight control, diet, and exercise
www.caloriecontrol.org

Centers for Disease Control and Prevention (CDC)
Atlanta, GA; 1–404–639–3311
www.cdc.gov

National Stroke Association
9707 E. Easter Lane
Englewood, CO 80112
1–800–STROKES
www.stroke.org

TOPS—TakePounds off Sensibly
http://www.tops.org/

The National Coalition for Women with Heart Disease—
WomenHeart http://www.womanheart.com/
phone: 202–728–7199

U.S. Department of Health and Human Services, Office on
Women's Health, National Women's Health Information Center
www.4woman.gov
800–994–WOMAN (9662)
TDD: 888–220–5446

Selected Books and Articles to Help You

1. *Using focus groups to develop a heart disease prevention program
for ethnically diverse, low-income women.* Gettleman L; Winkleby
MA J *Community Health (Journal of Community Health)* 2000
Dec; 25(6): 439–53 *Libraries Worldwide*: 643 (MEDLINE)

2. *Primary prevention programs to reduce heart disease risk in
women.* Halm MA; Denker J Source: *Clin Nurse Spec (Clinical
Nurse Specialist CNS.)* 2003 Mar; 17(2): 101–9; quiz 110–1
Libraries Worldwide: 691 (MEDLINE)

3. *Strategies for cardiovascular disease prevention: importance of
public and community health programs.* Egan BM; Lackland DT
Source: *Ethn Dis (Ethnicity & disease).* 1998; 8(2): 228–39
Libraries Worldwide: 126 (MEDLINE)

4. *Key elements for church-based health promotion programs: outcome-based literature review.* Peterson J; Atwood JR; Yates B Public *Health Nurs (Public Health Nursing).* 2002 Nov-Dec; 19(6): 401–11 *Libraries Worldwide:* 682 (MEDLINE)

5. Sandmaier, Marian. Healthy heart handbook for women [Bethesda, Md.] : U.S. Dept. of Health and Human Services, National Institutes of Health, National Heart, Lung, and Blood Institute, 2003.

6. Randall, Otelio S. and Donna Randall. "Menu for Life: African Americans get healthy, eat well, lose weight, and live beautifully." New York: Random House, 2003.

7. Nash, Jonell. "Low-Fat Soul." New York: Ballantine, 1996.

8. Keep the beat: Heart Healthy Recipes from the National Heart, Lung, and Blood Institute, U.S. Dept. of Health and Human Services, National Institutes of Health, National Heart, Lung, and Blood Institute, NIH Publication No. 03–2921, July 2003.

9. Castelli, William P. and Glen C. Griffin. "The new good fat bad fat: reduce your heart attack odds." Tucson: Fisher Books, 1989.

INDEX

144

INDEX